B[
always stood at the
BACK ! So that
she couldn't be
SPLASHED !!

THANKS for BUYING IT.
xxxxxxx
Philip E
12/9/90.
BM NORWICH

The Knee Joint:
A Clinical Guide

Philip Evans MBBS MRCS LRCP
Clinical Anatomist,
Clinical Assistant, Accident Unit,
Clinical Assistant, Orthopaedic Department,
The Norfolk and Norwich Hospital,
England

CHURCHILL LIVINGSTONE
EDINBURGH LONDON MELBOURNE AND NEW YORK 1986

CHURCHILL LIVINGSTONE
Medical Division of Longman Group Limited

Distributed in the United States of America by Churchill Livingstone,
Inc., 1560 Broadway, New York, N.Y. 10036, and by associated
companies, branches and representatives throughout the world.

First published 1986

ISBN 0-443-03248-3

British Library Cataloguing in Publication Data
Evans, Philip, *1935 July 7-*
  The knee joint: a clinical guide.
  1. Knee
  I. Title
  611'.72   QM131

Library of Congress Cataloging in Publication Data
Evans, Philip, M.B., B.S., M.R.C.S., L.R.C.P.
  The knee joint.
  Bibliography: p.
  Includes index.
  1. Knee.   2. Knee—Atlases.   I. Title.
  [DNLM: 1. Knee Joint—atlases.   WE 17 E921k]
  QM131.E93   1986   612'.75   85-17070

Produced by Longman Singapore Publishers (Pte) Ltd.
Printed in Singapore

Preface

The prime purpose of this book is to help anyone who has to deal with knee joints to improve the two essential clinical skills—taking a history and examining the joint. The section which explains the clinical tests is one aspect of this, but those parts which describe the workings of each component of the joint should lay the foundation for a deeper understanding of its mechanisms.

The book is designed as a post-graduate workbook, to be carried in the pocket and used on the couch, at the X-ray screen, or in short breaks. I hope it will find readers among junior and middle orthopaedic staff trying to improve their clinical diagnoses in the sports clinic or before arthroscopy, and physiotherapists, who wish to deepen their knowledge of functional anatomy when practising mobilisation or manipulation therapy. No excuse is needed for a book restricted to the workings of one joint, for the knee features largely in the workload of all physiotherapy, orthopaedic and accident departments.

However the viewpoint of the text is as much mechanical as medical, so that those readers with leanings towards biomechanics and bio-engineering, or even physical anthropology, will find here a description of the workings of a synovial joint that is hard to find outside the journals.

The drawings are designed for those who find pictures more helpful than words. Some readers may be unused to drawings without captions. For those it should be said that all clues to orientation are there in the drawings, and that the text can be seen as a running comment on the drawings, and vice versa. Indeed text and drawings are linked together throughout the book, facing each other almost always.

Relevant papers are constantly referred to in relation to text and drawings—this is intended to encourage the reader to enjoy the remarkable literature on this joint, and to base her or his clinical practice upon it. References are collected into a Bibliography, and their usage in the text is included in the Index. The short Glossary is designed for those less familiar with the argot of the subject—a perilous state sometimes!

Any feedback will be welcome, corrective or complimentary—after two thousand three hundred hours of working for the readers, it would be nice to know what they think of it. I hope, above all, that they will find it *useful*, that greater understanding will lead to better clinical practice, that in the end the ultimate beneficiary will be—the knee joint.

1986   P. J. Evans

Acknowledgements

It is a pleasure to thank those who have helped to ease the labour of producing this book.

My withdrawal from the social scene for weeks at a time over a number of years, was not only inconvenient but may at times have been felt somewhat as a personal slight. Family and friends suffered, we all suffered, and I hope that the appearance of a real book will do something to mitigate the loss of companionship and labour.

Next, Dinah Bagshaw and Mary Law of Churchill Livingstone, who used tact and restraint in teaching me the difference between the ideal aspired to and the worldly reality of commerce; and Ellen Green, who was both kind and perspicacious at the very beginning of this project. Thank you all for doing your job so well.

Next, those who have allowed me to use diagrams as bases for drawings in this book. To the editor of the *Journal of Bone and Joint Surgery* and to authors, thanks for allowing me to copy Fig 2a and 2b in Brantigan and Voshell (1941) for 8.12, and Fig 2 in Hughston et al (1976) for 9.1. To the editor of *Clinical Orthopaedics and Related Research* and to Fakhry Girgis of Cornell University Medical College and Peter S. Trent of the Hospital for Special Surgery in New York, thanks for allowing me to use Figs 6b, 7, and 15, from Girgis and Marshall (1975) for 9.3, 9.18, 9.7 & 9.8, and Figs 1 and 2 from Trent et al (1976) for 1.16 and 1.17. To the editor of the *British Journal of Bone and Joint Surgery* and to the author, thanks for allowing me to use Fig 2 from Wynne-Davies (1970) for 1.13. To Ronald McRae and Churchill Livingstone Publishers, thanks for allowing me to use Fig 83 on page 147 of *Clinical Orthopaedic Examination* (1976), for 2.32. To Dennis Stoker and Chapman and Hall Publishers, thanks for allowing me to make tracings of two radiographs in *Knee*

Arthrography (1982) for 4.4 and 4.5. To the Oxford University Press, thanks for allowing me to use Fig 161 from *Cunningham's Manual of Practical Anatomy* 13th edition (1969) for 8.16.

Many people have helped with the text as the book took shape over four years. Jill Guymer and Hugh Phillips both spent precious time applying their formidable talents to reading and making valued criticism. Robin Coupland, Jackie Critchley, Mike Fielding, Jane Heath, Sandra Mitchell, Graham Sneath, Jill Swain, Peter Wells and Sarah Williams all gave helpful advice from their standpoint as teachers or readers. John Cozens-Hardy's meticulous use of the English language helped me to re-draft part of the Preface. John MacNae helped with discussions of both text and clinical material, and was most supportive when time was needed to meet production deadlines. Thanks also go to Brenda Evans and Gillian my wife for their great help in checking the proofs. From Malcolm Glasgow and Hugh Phillips I have learnt an enormous amount about the orthopaedics of the knee. I thank them for all their teaching. Dominic, Simon and Paul, that cheerful trio, made smooth the passage of learning from the dissection of autopsy specimens.

Gray's Anatomy was used for reference several times, and Kapandji's *Physiology of the Joints* occasionally. The girls of the British Library at Boston Spa deserve a special vote of thanks for their superb service in providing reprints of articles, and Sue Bennett and associates in the Thomas Browne Library gave cheerful and efficient service, sometimes under difficulties.

Contents

one **Joint movements**

Introduction

The movements of the whole joint will first be described, then the way the articular surfaces travel over each other to produce those movements. The controlling mechanisms are next described, and finally there is a short section on the movements of the knee in standing, walking and running.

Movements of the joint

There are several ways of describing joint movements, viz. active and passive, physiological and accessory, conjunct and adjunct. To prevent difficulties, these will first be explained.

Physiological movements are voluntary (active) movements, such as flexion–extension and medial and lateral rotation. But they can also be performed by an examiner, i.e. passively. Accessory movements are those that only an examiner can make happen, like adduction and abduction (varus–valgus movements), A–P and P–A glides (the drawer movements), and occasionally transverse glide and compression–distraction movements. In biomechanical terms, the movements between the bones, such as roll, spin and glide, are also called accessory movements. *They* occur at the joint surfaces during physiological movements. Here they are covered in the section on movements of the articular surfaces, page 12 et seq.

Conjunct rotation is the phrase for an incidental amount of rotation that occurs during flexion and extension, as described below. Adjunct rotation is used for medial and lateral rotation as an independent movement as above, i.e. physiological rotations, either active or passive. The phrase 'adjunct rotation' is unfortunate though necessary, and is only used in textbooks or academic argument, when the two sorts of rotation need to be distinguished.

For a simple way of understanding knee movements, they are here presented under three headings: active movements, conjunct movements and passive movements.

Active movements

These are produced voluntarily by the muscles of the joint. The main voluntary movements of this hinge joint are, of course, flexion and extension (1.1). When the joint is in flexion, the tibia can be actively medially rotated and laterally rotated (1.2).

Conjunct movements

These 'happen with' other movements (Latin *conjunctus* = joined together), and are automatic and inevitable. As the knee comes up into extension there is a gradual conjunct lateral rotation of the tibia on the femur. This is easily seen in most people's knees, expecially in the last 20° of extension. It is seen best of all in a dissected joint. If the foot is fixed, as in the stance phase of walking, the femur medially rotates on the tibia.

So the knee movements of flexion–extension are thus not pure hinge movements, with a single sagittal axis (1.3), but are accompanied by a swivel (1.4). Conjunct rotation is nothing to do with muscles. It happens simply because of the mechanics of the joint, being present in a knee removed from a cadaver and stripped right down to bones, ligaments and menisci. See Trent et al (1976).

(Surprising things happen when you take time to really look at bones and joints. On the distal end of the femur, the grooves occupied by the fronts of the menisci in extension provide evidence for the conjunct rotation that occurs; see (1.5).)

Passive movements

These are knee movements produced by an examiner. Some are physiological movements produced passively, such as flexion–extension and medial and lateral rotation. Others are

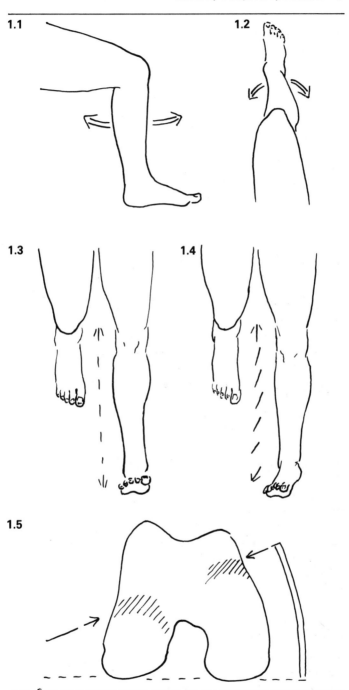

different, for in mechanical terms they are manoeuvres designed to reveal the working tolerance of the joint. These are called accessory movements. They are tests to reveal the amount of play available. They may reveal excessive play (laxity) or loss of normal play (stiffness), especially in the rotations. As physiological movements were covered above, only the accessory movements will now be described.

Rotational movements (adjunct rotation). In the passive (objective) examination of the knee, the tibia is medially and laterally rotated in flexion to check for stiffness or laxity; see (1.6) and (1.7). This 'winding up' of the joint into medial or lateral rotation may also effect the extent of anterior or posterior drawer movement, and is discussed in the section on clinical tests, page 148 et seq. It is also fully discussed in Slocum & Larson (1968) *Rotatory Instability of the Knee.*

Varus–valgus movements. When a knee is off-extension, some passive varus–valgus movement (or adduction–abduction) can be produced by the examiner. Normally, these passive movements cannot be found at full extension because the ligaments are tight—this is close-pack (pp. 124 and 126). But as flexion develops, and the joint goes into loose-pack, they can be produced. They cannot be performed by the patient; they can only be shown as the examiner strains the joint and overcomes the elasticity of the ligaments. See (1.8) and (1.9).

If the axis of flexion–extension is drawn as a dotted line (curved because of the conjunct rotation), this normal laxity on a transverse plane (or in rotations) can be represented as an area round the line, as at (1.10). This is called a joint perimeter. Again, note that there is normally no laxity in extension.

Generally, more adduction (varus) movement can be produced than abduction (valgus) movement. This shows that in (say) 20° of flexion, the lateral ligamentous complex is normally more lax than the medial complex. For varus and valgus stress tests, see pages 142 to 148, in the section on clinical tests.

Antero-posterior movements. These are the sagittal glides between the knee bones, known clinically as 'drawer movements'. The naming comes from the examination couch; see (1.11). Thus anterior drawer movement is anterior movement of the tibia under the femur: P–A glide. Posterior drawer movement is posterior movement of the tibia under the femur: A–P glide. Traditionally these movements test the

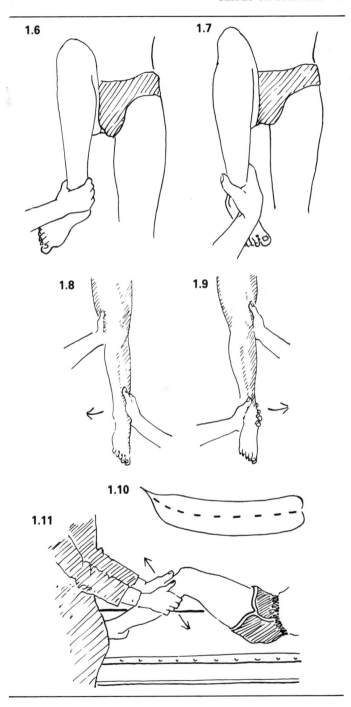

function of the cruciate ligaments, but they also test other structures as well; see ligament tests, pages 138–170. Gliding movements in the transverse plane are sometimes tried in an attempt to reproduce a patient's symptoms.

Compression and distraction. Compression of the patello-femoral joint is used both as a diagnostic aid and a therapeutic manoeuvre; see page 40. Distraction can have similar uses as well.

Combined movements. The combined movements of flexion–abduction–internal (tibial) rotation and flexion–adduction–external (tibial) rotation are sometimes known as 'quadrants'. A similar pair of combined movements near extension—extension–adduction and extension–abduction—complete the quartet of quadrants. They are marked with crosses in drawing (1.12), a schematic illustration of play in a joint, a movement perimeter.

Combined movements are the most searching form of passive movements in the passive (objective) examination, for they test the extremes of range of each type of movement in combination. They direct a high intensity stress on to the structures·of the joint, and especially on its ability to perform the slides and glides that are accessory to its normal range of movement (Guymer, 1984). Besides their importance as searching tests, they may elicit symptoms that are recognised by patients as their complaint, thus giving the therapist a guide for mobilisation therapy.

Range of active flexion-extension

Usually these are tested by the examiner as both passive and active movements. Normal passive range is from about 5° of hyper-extension or less to flexion where the heel is nearly in contact with the buttock. If there was 10° to 15° of hyper-extension, one would quickly look for other signs of joint laxity: see drawings here (1.13) from Wynne-Davis (1970); these are five generally accepted tests for generalised joint laxity. However, there may be a specific cause in the knee, *vide infra.*

Knee extension may be limited if the hip is anywhere beyond 90° flexion, as the hamstrings may become passively insufficient—'too short'.

1.12

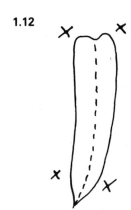

1.13

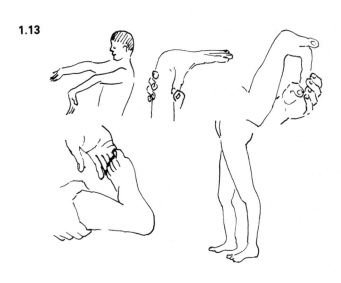

Axis of flexion-extension

The transverse axis for hinge movement varies. In full flexion it is well posterior on the femoral condyle, pretty well at the epicondyle (1.14). It is almost the same at 90° flexion. But as extension is approached the axis moves forwards. This is more fully discussed under 'shape of joint surfaces' on page 32.

The sagittal axis of flexion–extention changes through the movement because of conjunct rotation, for the femur is internally rotated in full extension and externally rotated in full flexion. (Or with a fixed femur, the tibia is externally rotated in full extension and internally rotated in full flexion.) See (1.15) and below, range and axis of conjunct movements.

Range of active rotatory movements

Not usually tested as such. Tested passively; see passive movements.

Axis of active rotatory movements

See under axis of passive rotatory movements.

Range and axis of conjunct movements

Conjunct rotation occurs throughout the range of hinge movement, but especially in the last 15° of extension, when it is known as the 'terminal screw-home of the knee'. As said above, it is a medial rotation of the femur if on a fixed tibia, or a lateral rotation of a free tibia under a fixed femur, as extension is approached.

Throughout the range of flexion there is some 40° of conjunct rotation (Trent et al, 1976). Half of it occurs in the 15° of movement up to extension. See (1.16) here. The range of conjunct rotation has been measured during walking—the knee rotates an average of 8° through stance phase; see Levens & Inman (1948) *Transverse Rotations of the Segments of the Lower Extremity in Locomotion*. But the range of flexion used in the stance phase of walking is surprisingly small—from about 10° flexion at heel-strike, to some 35° flexion at toe-off. (Swing phase needs 60° to 75° flexion; see walking and running, pp. 24 and 26.)

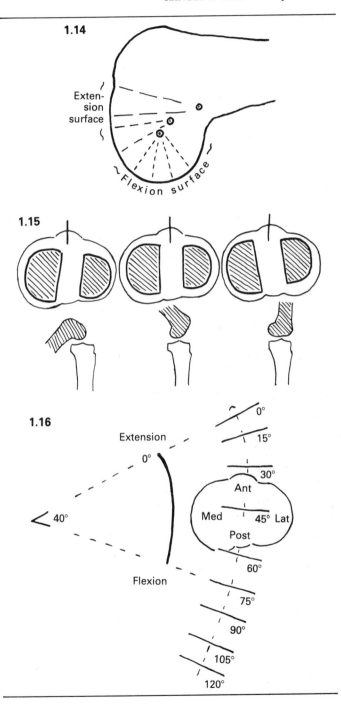

1.14

Extension surface

Flexion surface

1.15

1.16

Extension

0°

40°

Flexion

0°
15°
30°
Ant
Med   45° Lat
Post
60°
75°
90°
105°
120°

The axis of conjunct rotation has been nicely demonstrated by Trent et al in their 1976 paper. See (1.17) here, which is redrawn from their diagram with permission. It is around the back of the medial tibial spine, medial to it in the flexor range, and lateral to it near extension. See also pages 15, 121 and 165.

Range and axis of passive movements

When an examiner puts the joint into full extension to check for laxity, there should be no adduction–abduction movements possible, nor any anterior or posterior drawer movement (P–A or A–P glide). The ligaments are all tight, and no 'play' should be detectable. This is the close-packed state, more fully considered on page 124.

By 10° to 15° of flexion it is normal to be able to produce adduction and abduction movements. The range is usually around 10°, though adduction is generally more than abduction, with a looser 'feel'. This is because the lateral ligament is actually lax in flexion.

The effect is to produce a 'perimeter' of passive joint movements found on examination that looks like (1.18). Laxity of the anterior and central part of the medial ligament would give a perimeter shape as in (1.19).

Axis of passive rotations. This is similar to the axis of conjunct rotation (above), being around the posterior end of the medial tibial spine. The ranges of rotation are usually around 25° to 30°.

Drawer movements. Despite the large amount of research papers, the anterior and posterior drawer tests remain manual and clinical tests. It is the hand and the eye together that assess the direction, amount, and feel of tibial movement. The only attempt at measurement is to compare it with the opposite side. In experienced hands, this seems to work well.

Let us take, for example, the anterior drawer test. Its range can be learned by experience, and the direction. The 'feel' is the difference between a rapidly diminishing elasticity over a short range, in the normal, and an absolute laxity over a longer range with a rapid but soft stop at the end, in the abnormal. The first is simply stretching the anterior cruciate and medial ligaments; the second is almost free movement forwards of the tibia, but brought up short by the back of the femoral condyles riding up on the posterior parts of the menisci. See (1.20) and (1.21).

1.17

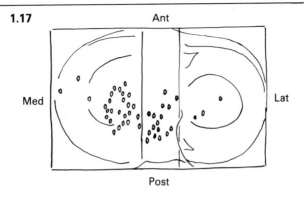

Ant

Med

Lat

Post

1.18

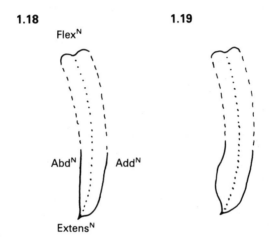

Flex^N

Abd^N Add^N

Extens^N

1.19

1.20

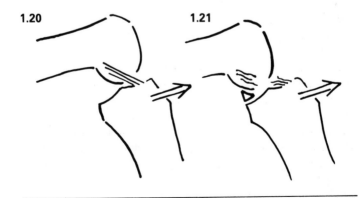

1.21

Movements of the articular surfaces

Introduction

Between the surfaces articulating, movement occurs either as a roll, a glide, or a spin. But there is no real spin in the knee, despite its ability to rotate. For during an active movement of rotation-in-flexion (that is, adjunct rotation), the axis lies more between the condyles of the femur than under one of them. So they glide in opposite directions, the lateral condyle more than the medial one; see below. The main movements are gliding and rolling, and these terms will be brought in as part of the description of the movements of the areas in contact.

Movements at the articular surfaces

The areas in contact are here called the articulation patches. The medial patch is bigger than the lateral patch, by about a third (Walker & Hajek, 1972, p. 583). On the tibia, the articulation patches consist of a roundish area of tibial surface with a rim of meniscal surface outside it.

At the femur. On the femoral surface, the patches move from posterior in flexion to anterior in extension; see (1.22). The articulation patches are smaller in flexion than in extension, chiefly because of the greater curvature of the flexor surface (1.22, 1.23, 1.24). But additionally on the lateral side, the femoral surface is norrower from side to side at the flexor end; see (1.25).

In moving from flexion to extension, from the back of the tibia to the front, the motion at the surface of the femur is in large part a rolling motion. (But rather more of a slide on the medial side; see later.) However a moment spent measuring the surfaces reveals that the appropriate surface available on the femur is about 6 cm long, whereas that on the tibia is about 4.5 cm long. Thus there must be a considerable element of backwards sliding of the femoral surface upon the meniscus and tibia in addition to the roll, as the joint moves from flexion to extension. At the articular surfaces, therefore, there is both rolling and sliding motion.

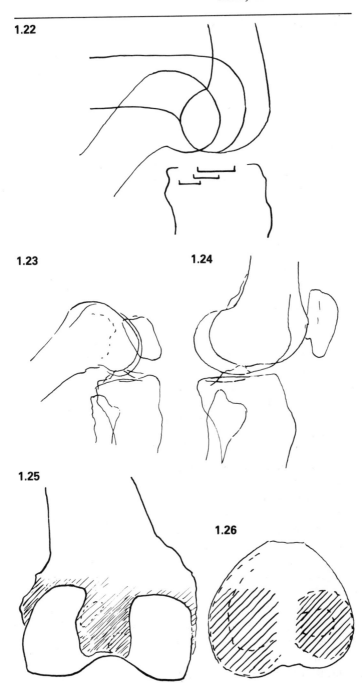

1.22

1.23   1.24

1.25

1.26

At the tibia and menisci. As on the femur, the medial contact patch is always larger than the lateral one; see (1.26). Hence the larger size of the entire medial tibial plateau—see (2.17) and (2.18).

Taking first the movement from full flexion to 20° flexion, the two tibial patches are again more posterior in flexion, and more anterior near extension. This shift is much more marked on the lateral side—see schematic diagram (1.27). The appearance is as if the transverse axis is fixed near the medial border of the joint (perhaps at the proximal attachment of the medial ligament?), so that the lateral patch moves in an arc (1.28). (See also de Peretti et al (1983, p. 6.) This is the arc of conjunct rotation, diagram (1.16). On the lateral side, the meniscus moves with its femoral condyle, sliding over the tibia as the femur rolls and slides upon it. On the medial side, the meniscus moves but little between full flexion and 20°; here the femoral movement is mostly a slide.

Between some 20° of flexion and full extension, a change takes place. The medial articulation patch moves back as well, thus increasing the rate of conjunct rotation. See (1.29)—very schematic. At the same time the more flattened profile of the femoral condyle at its extensor surface (1.30) leads to a general enlargement of the articulation patches, especially antero-posteriorly. The menisci, previously opened out transversely (1.31), become stretched more antero-posteriorly (1.32). Their anterior parts are closely held between femur and tibia in full extension, and they groove both surfaces. The femur especially shows these markings well (1.33 and 1.34); on some femora the complete medial meniscal shape may be seen—perhaps these were soldiers or barbers, or surgeons!

The more anterior grooving of the medial condyle reflects its movement posteriorly as extension is approached—the terminal conjunct rotation in extension.

Limitations of movement

Movement may be limited for many reasons, some of which are covered here:

(i) Articular surface problems. Chondromalacia, loss of articular cartilage from osteo-arthritis. Different 'feel' of slide and glide, compression may give pain. Range of movement can be full.

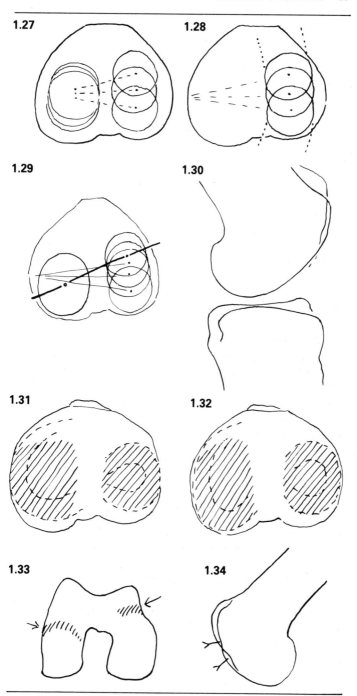

(ii) Impingement of aberrant material between articular surfaces, such as part of a torn meniscus, a loose body from osteochondritis dissecans, or a swollen fat pad. Loss of range, with abnormal end-feel. Patient may localise the problem place. Commonest is the old-age loss of range, with bony build-up at the edges of articular surfaces.

(iii) Muscle shortening or skin contracture. Cerebral palsy, fibrous scar in rectus femoris, burns on the extensor surface. Alteration of one range of movement only. Patient may localise the cause. Actual joint not involved.

(iv) Contracted scar tissue in the capsule or soft tissue close round the joint. An example is a twisted ankle with extensive bruising, that has been immobilised too long. Loss of range in all movements, with different end-feel. Changes in accessory movements such as glides and passive rotations.

(v) Haemarthrosis and effusion, with or without muscle spasm. Simple traumatic effusion, mild sprain medial complex, avulsion fracture anterior cruciate origin. Movements very limited, sometimes impossible. Not easy—sorts out the sheep from the goats! See page 138, The acute knee, and Effusions, page 82.

(vi) Pain in the knee. Cause may be inside the joint, often with limitation of movement, or outside it, often with full range of movement. In the first category, torn meniscus, loose body, OA patella; in the second, iliotibial tract friction syndrome, inflamed pre-patellar bursa, and irritable hip. A full history with an understanding of knee joint mechanisms is essential, giving 70% of diagnoses. The examination must include firm palpation with the thumb to find the tender spot.

Excessive movement—joint laxity

(i) Changes in the joint surface, such as loss of articular cartilage (Rh. A, O.A.,), or depressed fracture of lateral tibial condyle. The ligaments are left 'too long'.

(ii) Familial joint laxity or hypermobility.

(iii) Excessive length of constraining structures, e.g. trauma to medial ligament and anterior cruciate, or destruction of cruciates by Rh. A.

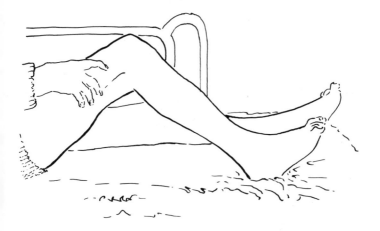

Control of knee movements

Stabilising the bones

At first sight the arrangement of the ligaments may appear somewhat random; see (1.35). However, some generalisations are applicable:

(i) Their femoral attachments are on or near a line joining the epicondyles viz., near the line of the transverse axis in flexion. The diagram (1.36) shows that the two cruciates are attached very close to the axis, and the medial and lateral collateral ligaments and the arcuate (postero-lateral) complex are almost on the axis. In (1.35) the ligaments are drawn on to an X-ray tracing.

(ii) The central pair resist internal tibial rotation (external rotation of the femur), and the peripheral group resist external tibial rotation (internal rotation of the femur). This can be derived from diagram (1.36).

(iii) Each femoral condyle is on a short (internal) rein and a long (external) rein.

With reference to (i) above, all the ligaments will tend to become tensed if the epicondyle lifts off the tibial surface—as happens when full extension is achieved from 20° flexion. See also Joint Surfaces—femur, page 32.

Referring now to (ii) above, on the medial side of the joint—see (1.37) and (1.38)—the medial ligament prevents anterior tibial glide and external tibial rotation (Brantigan & Voshell, 1941) and the posterior cruciate prevents posterior tibial glide (and possibly internal tibial rotation). On the lateral side of the joint—see (1.38) and (1.39)—the fibular collateral and the arcuate complex prevent posterior tibial glide and external tibial rotation; the anterior cruciate prevents anterior tibial glide and internal tibial rotation.

Clinically, medial ligament damage is linked with anterior cruciate damage, for both resist anterior glide, as well as pure abduction. Similarly, the posterior cruciate is clinically linked with the postero-lateral complex, as these all resist posterior glide strains, and adduction. Damage from rotary strains is variable; it can be surprisingly severe. See Hughston et al (1976), and Brantigan & Voshell (1941) again.

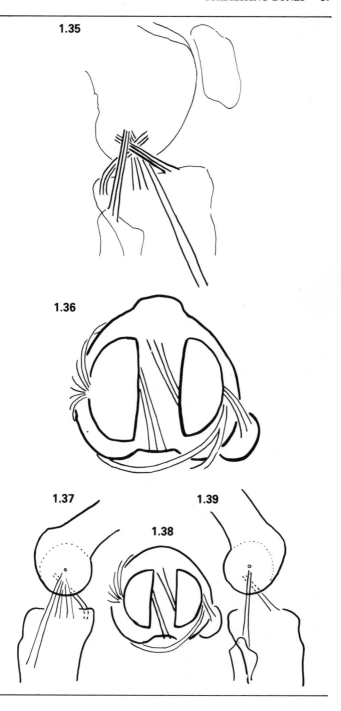

Controlling the axes of movement

The axis upon which the knee becomes stabilised will depend on the 'pull' from its ligaments. The 'pull' of a ligament varies according to the amount of increase in length available in those parts of the ligaments in tension. As the transverse (hinge) axis varies through flexion, and as the femoral attachments of a ligament may be 'off centre' anyway (e.g. the cruciates), then parts of a ligament will tend to become tensed or stretched if its femoral attachment becomes lifted away from its tibial origin. The collagen-elastin of ligaments can stretch by about 8% before tearing. Short ligaments like the central pair of cruciates (3.0 to 3.8 cm long) can lengthen say 0.25 cm before giving way. Peripheral ligaments like the oblique popliteal, fibular collateral, and medial ligament proper, being from 5 to 10 cm long, can lengthen by 0.4 to 0.8 cm before failure.

Thus in the last 20° of the movement towards extension, when the lift of the femoral epicondyles from the tibial surface is tensing all the ligaments, the cruciates become able to stretch no more, and the peripheral ligaments have to 'give'. So the cruciates draw the joint into medial rotation of the femur (lateral rotation of the tibia) as the knee comes up into extension. Their inability to further increase in length causes the terminal screw-home movement of the knee in full extension. This screw-home does not occur in the absence of the controlling ligaments. Thus without the anterior cruciate and postero-lateral complex, the lateral condyle is not drawn forward, and can be made to demonstrate the 'pivot-shift' test. This test is described on pages 160–169.

The closed kinematic chain

Each ligament varies in length from knee to knee—for instance Girgis et al (1975, p. 220) gives a variation of 40% for each cruciate in 24 knees. But work by the author on 10 knees indicates that when the ratios between the ligaments (and the bony dimensions) is measured, the figures are much more constant (Evans, 1985, *Annals of the Royal College of Surgeons (England)* 67, (3):196. The ratios were ACL 1.3 to 1, PCL 1.5 to 1, FCL 2.5 to 1, where 1 was the radius of their lateral femoral condyle in the flexor surface, on a lateral X-ray.

1.40

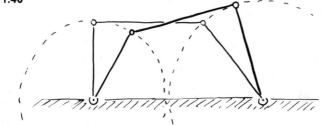

This harmony of proportion in the joint would be expected, since everything is related to everything else. But it also provides convincing evidence to support other workers' papers (e.g. Struben, 1982), that the joint acts as a 'closed kinematic chain'. This is a simple mechanical concept (1.40) of which the best-known example is the wheels and couplings of a steam locomotive; see (1.41). The connections have a length that is determined by their attachments to the moving parts. Or, the path of their attachments is determined by their length. See drawings of the medial and lateral halves of the joint, drawn in those terms (1.42) and (1.43).

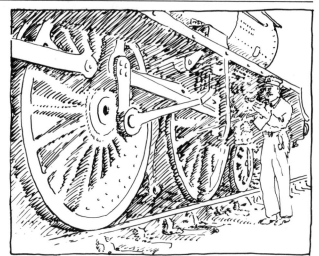

1.41

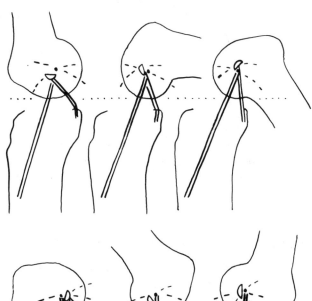

1.42

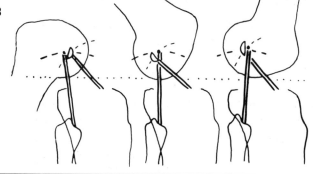

1.43

Standing, walking and running

Standing

The standing position may be either symmetrical or asymmetrical (Smith, 1953); see (1.44) and (1.45). In (1.44) the knees are neither extended nor flexed. Surprisingly there is no need for muscle power in the anti-gravity muscles, for the vertical line of the centre of gravity passes in front of the transverse axis of the knee, preventing flexion from occurring. See Akerblom (1948).

In (1.45) the weight-bearing limb is hyper-extended, being thrust back into the 'locked' or closely-packed position. The other limb rests on the ground as a steadier, being usually placed on a line passing transversely through the weight-bearing foot. The pelvic tilt that invariably accompanies (1.45) is a mechanism for tensing the iliotibial tract. The pull of the tract stabilises the knee in extension, as well as helping to resist extension and adduction at the hip (Evans, 1979).

The locking of asymmetrical standing is not the locking or jamming that occurs with a torn meniscus or loose body. It is normal, physiological locking, the subject of Barnett's 1953 paper. It is close-pack (see p. 12), which can happen in any joint. The holding of the joint into extension by the line of the centre of gravity is an over-centre device, like the collateral folding hinges of a dispatch case that snap back to hold the lid open.

Walking (see Saunders et al, 1953)

The knee is never in extension during walking. Through swing phase it is flexed between 60° and 75°, helping to lift the toes clear of the ground. Heel strike marks the beginning of stance phase, and here stability is paramount. The joint is held just flexed, at around 15°, with all the muscles active for stability; see (1.46). The ligaments will also be fairly tense, as the knee is close to extension. The joint thus has a high proportion of each stability factor in operation, viz. muscles strongly active, ligaments tense, and joint surfaces greatly congruent and bearing over a large area.

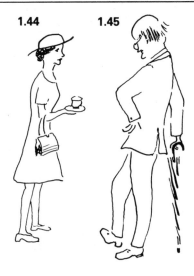

1.44   **1.45**

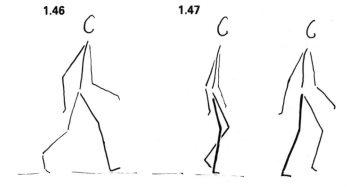

1.46   **1.47**

The knee flexes to about 20° as it passes beneath the body at mid-stance-phase (see 1.48), after which flexion decreases again—this prevents the body from bobbing up and down excessively. Energy is thus conserved by keeping the path of the centre of gravity as smooth as possible.

But shortly after the foot passes under the body, the heel lifts to initiate push-off (1.49). This would lengthen the limb (by adding on the length of the foot), so the knee flexes to compensate. The end of stance phase is toe-off, and here the knee is in considerable flexion (some 40°) both to compensate for the extra limb length added by the lifted foot, and to shorten the limb for swing phase, to help prevent the toes from dragging (1.50).

The generally flexor position adopted by the knee reduces body height—'. . . a person is slightly shorter when he is walking than when he is standing . . .' (Saunders et al, 1953, p. 545).

Running

During running, mobility becomes all-important. Smaller areas of the joint articulate, and stability is achieved as much by muscles as by ligaments. There is a general shift towards flexion. Thus at heel strike (which is probably actually toe strike) the knee is in considerable flexion, and throughout stance phase the knee is flexed more than in walking.

The biggest difference is in the forward swing. After the tremendous thrust of toe-off (1.51), the foot is flicked upwards as the thigh swings forwards (1.52). The knee becomes considerably flexed, and may be at 120° to 150° of flexion as it comes forward (1.53). The usefulness of this flexion is undoubted, for it has a simple and marvellous effect: by shortening the limb (at that time acting as a pendulum), less energy is required to swing it forward, fast.

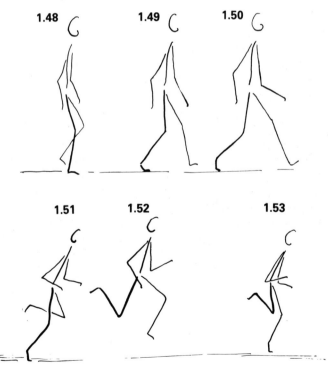

two Joint surfaces

Introduction

To get the best from this text you should have with you the following things: (i) a matching set of bones, femur, tibia and patella, preferably right-sided; (ii) two or three sets of X-rays of the knee, A-P and lateral, best obtained from the pile of time-expired films; (iii) a book or atlas that shows the soft tissue anatomy. The first two are more important than the third.

There are really two joints in the knee. (i) The patello-femoral joint, the joint of the extensor muscles. Symptoms from this joint appear especially with anti-gravity efforts—stairs and chairs, baths and cars. (ii) The knee joint proper, between femur and tibia and the menisci. This is the joint of functional weightbearing. Thus its symptoms are usually found in the stance phase of walking or running.

Even the knee joint proper is best seen as having two parts. The upper surface of the menisci is for flexion-extension and the lower surface for axial rotation. Or to simplify, the curves of the femoral condyles move in the hollows of the menisci in flexion-extension, while the flat under-surfaces of the menisci move on the tibial plateau in rotation. Of course it is more complicated than that, but the generalisation is fair.

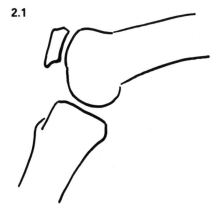

2.1

Femoral surfaces for tibia and menisci

The femur, anterior view

The distal end of the femur articulates both with the patella and with the tibio-meniscal surface. Looking at the bone, the two articular areas can be distinguished because they are separated by slight indentations. Though not always easily seen, these mark where the anterior part of each meniscus is squeezed between tibia and femur in full extension. See (2.2), where the meniscal grooves are hatched.

With the knee flexed, an A-P view shows the femoral condyles to be curved, rounded off as if to run like wheels between the tibial spines centrally and the meniscal rim periferally (2.3). The deep hollow between the bearing surfaces is for the cruciate ligaments. Look at an A-P X-ray and (i) try and work out where the menisci are; (ii) notice the difference between the medial and the lateral bearing surface of the femur. Both become less rounded in extension, and more rounded in flexion (2.4).

The femur, lateral view

A side view of the dry bone again shows the shallow meniscal groove that separates the anterior patellar surface from the tibio-meniscal surface; see (2.5) and (2.6). Take the lateral X-ray and define the two surfaces. Then distinguish lateral and medial femoral condyles. Even if its groove is too faint, the medial one usually exhibits the hillock of the adductor tubercle (for adductor magnus) where the shaft joins the condyle behind. The lateral one merely has a notch there.

2.2

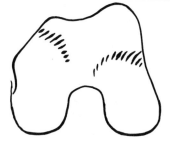

2.3

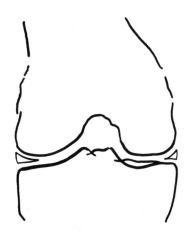

2.4

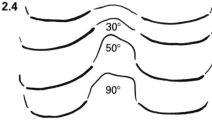

30°

50°

90°

2.5

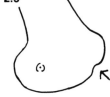

2.6

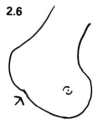

Now draw round the outline of the bone; mark in the meniscal groove and the epicondyle (where the collateral ligament attaches). Make measurements to establish the radius of curvature, and mark in the radii at various angles. This is a revealing exercise; see (2.7) and (2.8).

If the patellar surface is disregarded, the lateral view of the femoral articular surface can be seen either as (i) a flat for extension plus a round for flexion, or (ii) a wheel and a wedge or (iii) a spiral. See the sketches (2.9)–(2.11) The measurements of radii show that this is how the ends of each ligament become forced apart as the joint comes up into extension. Note also how there is greater area of contact between joint surfaces in extension; i.e. in full extension the surfaces are maximally congruent (2.12). This is the close-packed condition of the joint.

Meniscal surfaces

The femur articulates with the menisci and the upper tibia, the menisci covering much of the area (2.13). The menisci have hollow upper surfaces (for the femur) and flat lower surfaces for the tibia (2.14). Though the meniscal cartilages are covered more fully later, this section looks at them in relationship to the femoral and tibial articular surfaces.

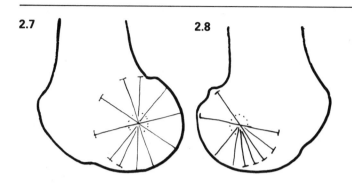

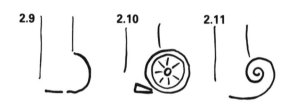

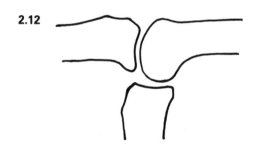

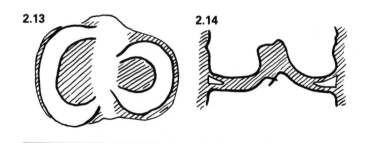

As the bearing surfaces of the femur are different in flexion to what they are in extension (see side view (2.7 and 2.8) the surface underneath should change too. What happens is that the femur bears more on the back of the tibial plateau in flexion, drawing the meniscus back with it (2.15). In extension the contact area moves anteriorly (2.16). The menisci become squashed out to an oval in extension as the femoral bearing profile changes.

Anterior views also reveal how the femoral bearing profile changes from flexion through to extension. See the bone and (2.4). Again, the bearing surface is more rounded in flexion and less rounded in extension. Again, the tibia and menisci must match these changes.

Tibial surfaces for femur and menisci

Take the bone, and looking down on the tibial plateau, confirm the following:

(i) The medial and lateral halves are off-set from the sagittal midline of the shaft (2.17). Possible reason: the medial femoral rotation that occurs at the knee in full extension.

(ii) The medial surface is larger than the lateral surface. Possible reason: the greater weight carried through the medial compartment.

(iii) Both surfaces exhibit markings that separate meniscal areas (peripheral) from femoral areas (central); see (2.18). Find the facets that mark the attachment of the horns of the menisci; check with the hatched areas in sketch (2.18). Distinguish them from those made by the cruciate ligaments, dotted outline in sketch (2.18).

(iv) On the medial side, the surface for direct contact with the femur is bi-concave, i.e. scooped out. On the lateral side it is concave seen from anterior, but convex seen from the side; it is saddle-shaped. (2.19). Possible reason: for medial stability, but lateral mobility. See de Peretti et al (1983).

(v) The medial tibial spine is a long, low hump; the lateral spine is a short high peak (2.22). Possible reason: long A-P medial contact area; small, mobile lateral contact area.

(vi) Now look from the front and the side (2.20) The two articular surfaces are not parallel; they are off-set like the

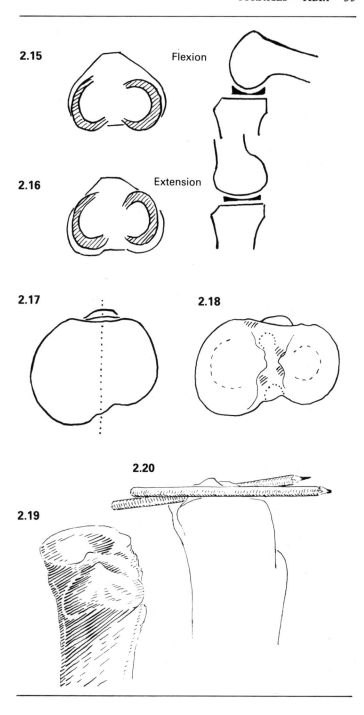

2.15 Flexion

2.16 Extension

2.17

2.18

2.20

2.19

blades of a twin propeller. Possible reason: connected to the rotation in terminal extension.

(vii) The differing contours of the medial and lateral tibial plateaux are confirmed on the front view (2.21) and the side view (2.22). Note how the lateral profile seems to run right off the edge both posteriorly and anteriorly. This 'run-off' is for the lateral meniscus in extreme flexion and maximum extension. Contrast with the back of the medial plateau—sharp and overhanging.

Now examine some lateral X-rays and try and read the medial and lateral articular surfaces of the tibia and their spines. The two femoral condyles were distinguished earlier, on page 30. A typical X-ray is outlined here (2.23). Others are (2.25), (3.1) and (9.4).

See also Danzig et al (1981) Osseous Landmarks of the Normal Knee. This is a well-made paper about reading the medial and lateral surfaces of tibia and femur on an X-ray, leading to a way of spotting dislocation of the superior tibio-fibular joint. See also de Peretti et al (1983).

Patello-femoral surfaces

The sequence here is first the patella, then the femur, and then the mechanics of the joint. A good general source is the book by Ficat & Hungerford (1977).

The patella

The anterior surface of the patella is strongly marked by the quadriceps tendon. It does not concern us. The posterior surface articulates with the femur, and here the articular cartilage shows facets for the lateral and medial femoral condyles, each of which has separate areas for flexion and extension. See (2.15) here, and Hungerford & Barry (1979). This is thickest cartilage in the body (5–6 mm).

The lateral area is much larger than the medial area, which is appropriate to the mechanics of the joint; see page 44. There is also an 'odd' facet, a cartilage facet that is not always seen on the dry bone, which is only apposed in extreme flexion; see (2.24) again.

2.21

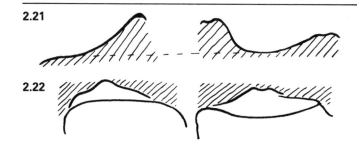

2.22

2.23

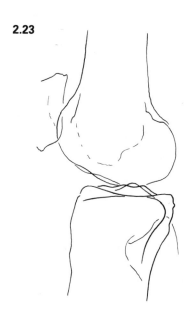

2.24

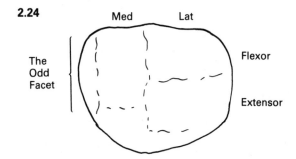

Med   Lat

The
Odd
Facet

Flexor

Extensor

Movements and articulation

As flexion proceeds, the patella slips distally in the femoral trochlea, whilst bending backwards on its tendon to become closer to the tibial plateau. See figure (2.25) here. This movement explains the presence of the deep infra-patellar bursa (5.10) Seen from the front, the track of the patella is C-shaped, open laterally. In extremes of flexion, the patella spins on the axis of the tendon slightly, moving in the trochlea so that the posterior surface faces somewhat laterally (2.27).

In extension, the patella lies on a fat pad proximal to the trochlea. As flexion begins, the patella engages with the lateral trochlear wall before the medial wall, then is embraced by both. The course of the articular patch was neatly demonstrated by Goodfellow et al's work in their first 1976 paper. It is a roughly dumb-bell-shaped area on both femur and patella, which moves, as flexion proceeds, down the trochlea and up the patella. See (2.26) and (2.28). As far as 90° of flexion, the medial and lateral patellar facets only are engaged. The odd facet (2.24) only comes into apposition in extreme flexion, as the patella rotates about a vertical axis; the odd facet then engages the lateral (inner) part of the flexed medial femoral condyle. See (2.27) and (2.28).

Looking at the femur, we should note that the dumbell patch moves in extreme flexion on to tibiomeniscal territory, viz. posterior to the meniscal grooves; see (2.29). This could be significant in linking patello-femoral disease with medial compartment disease; see below.

Clinical significance

The clinical test of posterior compression of the patella, if performed in extension, will not test the subchondral bone of the trochlea. For that the knee should be in flexion, say 60° if the pain comes when climbing stairs, or say 130° if it is painful to squat down.

The significance of the odd facet is brought out in Goodfellow's first 1976 paper and in Hungerford & Barry's paper of 1979. It is said that degeneration in this facetal surface is due to lack of use, the facet only engaging at more than 90° flexion, which doesn't happen often in a day. Since articular cartilage needs regular compression and wiping with fresh synovial fluid, the vital sweep and squeeze requirement is perhaps too infrequent. Compare hip joint degeneration in Bullough et al (1973).

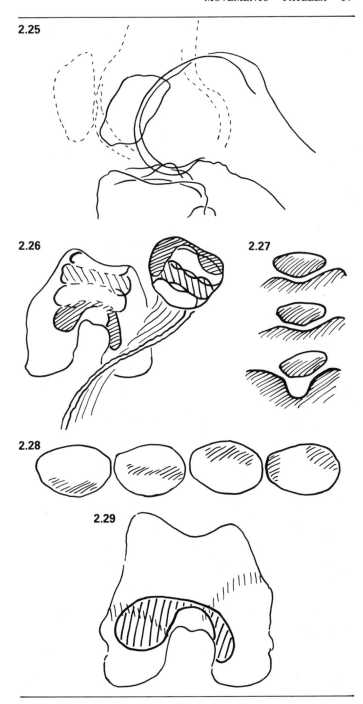

2.25

2.26

2.27

2.28

2.29

Goodfellow et al also postulated the link between surface degeneration in the odd facet and osteochondritis of the medial femoral condyle, which occurs just at the 'kissing point' of the odd facet. See (2.30) and (2.31).

Clinical aspects. See Insall (1982) *Patellar pain*

Although the deep surface of the patella is covered with the greatest thickness of articular cartilage in the body, it can still present as a clinical problem. A hard knock on the patella can cause direct injury to the cartilage (dashboard injury) from which it sometimes never recovers and which can lead to early osteoarthritis.

The term chondromalacia patellae is still used commonly as a clinical diagnosis. The author agrees with Goodfellow et al (1976a) that it should be used as a descriptive term for the appearance of the articular cartilage, adegenerative state secondary to some other cause. It may be found with painful syndromes such as abnormal tracking or malalignment (see later), or may be asymptomatic, being merely an incidental finding due to aging. See Goodfellow et al (1976b).

Patellar pain is probably linked to excessive point pressure on the subchondral bone; some athletes present with a painful over-use syndrome that is probably due to trabecular micro-fractures in the subchondral bone. Localised pain at the lower pole of the patella, where the patellar tendon joins the patella, can be due to repeated small avulsions of collagen from bone. This is 'jumper's knee', a similar pathology to tennis elbow.

The articular surface is accessible to palpation if the knee is extended and relaxed. Gentle medial displacement of the patella lifts up the medial edge, and the fingers can exert pressure directly on the medial facet, (2.32).

The characteristic stiffness in the knee after prolonged sitting probably reflects increased friction due to surface changes in the patellar hyaline cartilage. Pain in the extremes of flexor range, such as on squatting, would coincide with impingement of degeneration in the odd facet with the central part of the medial femoral condyle.

Medial facet pain is common in the young adolescent and young adult, and may be linked with chondromalacia patellae.

2.30

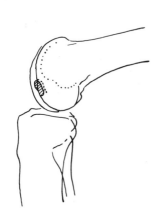

2.31

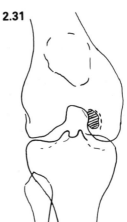

2.32

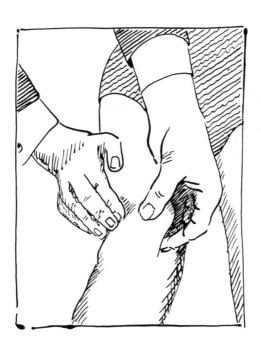

Lateral facet pain occurs commonly in osteoarthritis. Rough or raised joint margins may be palpated clinically. Radiography of the patellofemoral joint may show loss of joint space and peripheral osteophytes, confirming clinical judgement (2.33 and 2.34).

The compression load on the P–F joint is eight times the body weight in deep knee bends and three times body weight on stairs (Hungerford & Barry, 1979). If a patient gets pain in these activities, the patello-femoral joint should be a prime suspect. *NB*. Downstairs is often worse than up.

Patello-femoral joint surfaces —the femur

On the femur, the surface for the patella is separated from the surface for the tibia by slight indentations. These grooves are visible on the dry femur on both medial and lateral condyles; see drawing (2.35). They mark where the anterior part of the meniscus is squeezed between femur and tibia in full extension (2.37). A line roughly joining the grooves becomes yet another indicator of the rotation that occurs in full extension; see (2.36).

The lateral groove shows nicely on a lateral X-ray; by it the lateral condyle can be identified (2.38). It is less easy to see the groove on the medial condyle, though a search anteriorly may be rewarded.

Turning now to the deep groove for the patella, if you look directly up at the femoral condyle from distally you will see that the lateral lip of the patellar groove is much more prominent than the medial lip (2.35). This structural fact is linked with the mechanics of extensor pull across this joint. To understand this is to understand dislocation of the patella and how it is treated. Here is a brief explanation.

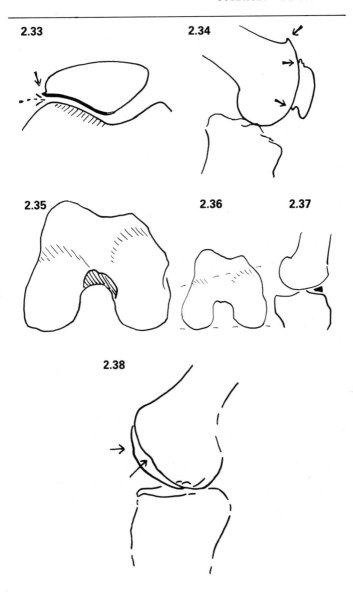

2.33

2.34

2.35

2.36

2.37

2.38

Keeping the patella in its place

Seen from in front, the hinge of the knee joint is straight across the tibia, but obliquely across the femur; see diagram (2.39). The reason for this is rooted in our mammalian ancestry and our upright posture: the pelvis is wide enough for the passage of a baby's head; the hip joint has a ball and socket of appropriate size; the femur has a neck for abductor leverage when upright. So a vertical drop from the greater trochanter would place the feet 15 in to 18 in apart: see (2.40).

But one of the ways we save energy when walking is by moving the centre of gravity forward with minimal up-and-down movement and minimal side-to-side movement. (See Saunders et al, (1953). The major determinants in normal and pathological gait—this is a wonderful paper.) So it is best if the feet are close together and the hinge joint of the knee has a nearly antero-posterior excursion. Hence the necessity for the obliquity of the femurs (2.41). Hence the *angle* between the femur and the tibia at the knee joint, called the 'physio-logical valgus'. And hence the anatomical description, 'the medial femoral condyle is longer than the lateral condyle'. See (2.43).

With quadriceps arising chiefly from the femur, its pull, like the shaft of the femur, is oblique to vertical, (2.44). But the patellar tendon must be nearly vertical for a horizontal hinge joint, so there is a mechanical tendency for the patella to slip laterally. Some might say, 'Vector analysis indicates a marked lateral component'. The angle between the pull of the quadriceps and the patellar tendon is known by clinicians as the 'Q' angle (2.45). The 'Q' angle is usually greater in women because of the greater breadth of the pelvis. 'Q' probably stands for Quadriceps.

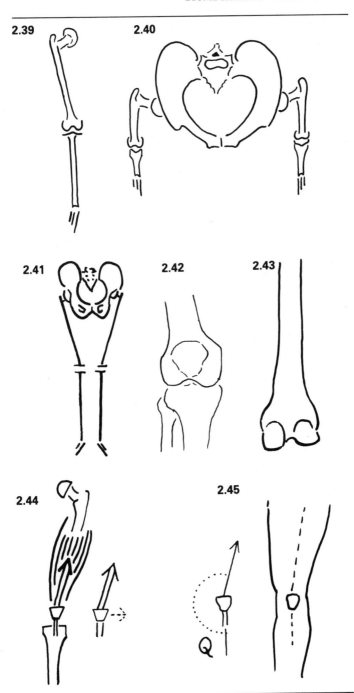

2.39

2.40

2.41

2.42

2.43

2.44

2.45

The tendency for the patella to slip laterally is resisted by bony, muscular and ligamentous structures (2.46).

(i) The high lateral wall of the patellar groove provides lateral resistance.

(ii) The lowest fibres of vastus medialis provide an active medial pull.

(iii) The medial fibres of the patellar retinaculum provide a passive resistance to lateral displacement.

Note that the most dangerous period for dislocation of the patella is near full extension; this is when the patella is losing the support of the lateral buttress of the femur. This is the time when vastus medialis muscle must be most active.

Clinical aspects (see Kettlecamp (1981) *Malalignment*)

The factors predisposing to dislocation of the patella are:

(i) Malalignment of tibia and femur. Anteversion of the neck of the femur, or internal rotation of the shaft of the femur, will produce squint patellae—inward-looking patella (2.48). The tibia turns outwards and prevents the feet pointing in, so there is an increase in the 'Q' angle. Genu valgum has a similar effect on the 'Q' angle.

(ii) Patello-femoral dysplasia. This usually presents as a small high patella (patella alta) with or without a low lateral femoral buttress.

(iii) Abnormalities of supporting structures. There can be tightness of the lateral patellar retinaculum or an abnormal tethering band from the iliotibial tract causing lateral tracking or lateral subluxation (2.50). Vastus medialis can be ineffective, or the medial retinacular structures weak as part of a generalised joint laxity (Fig. 1.13).

(iv) Trauma—a normal patella can be dislocated laterally by a sudden blow near extension. The medial ligamentous supports will have been torn.

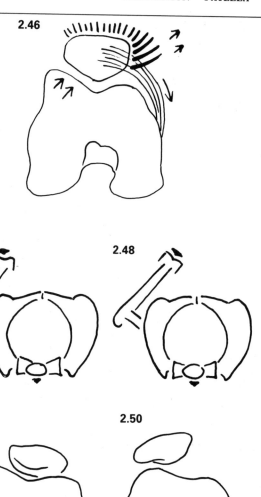

Clinical tests

The 'Patellar apprehension test' is used to see if a recent painful episode was in fact a dislocation or subluxation of the patella—they are not always easy to detect. On a couch, the knee is put in very slight flexion. The finger now quickly forces the patella laterally (2.51). Strong apprehension, or even physical restraint by the patient, constitutes a positive test: especially so if the sensation mimics their original symptoms.

There is a simple test for an abnormal tethering band from the iliotibial tract (personal communication, Hugh Phillips, 1984). With the patient supine, the patella is fingered to ensure it is loose above the femoral sulcus in extension. Then the limb is fully adducted at the hip, keeping the knee extended. The patella is again checked to see if it will still move from side to side (2.53). Failure to move medially in adduction points to a tethering band from the iliotibial tract, provided that quadriceps is not tense. See Ober (1935) and Jeffreys (1963). Ober's test (Ober, 1936) is for contracted iliotibial tract in cases of back pain caused by contraction of the upper iliotibial tract.)

Patellar tracking: The knee is flexed and extended, first actively then passively, while a close watch is kept upon the patella (2.52). Its excursion should be smooth, with no sudden jerks or flicks. It may jerk sideways, or rotate, and this may be more easily felt than seen.

For a very personal demonstration of patellar tracking, see the extraordinary letter by Austin (1981).

2.51

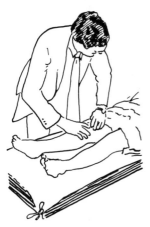

2.52

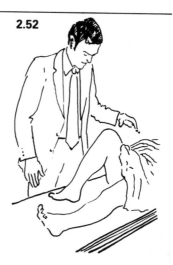

2.53

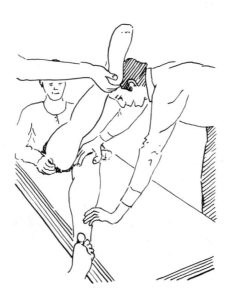

three **Articular cartilage**

Tibial surfaces

Hyaline articular cartilage forms the bearing surface of the joint. It is best visualised by a double contrast arthrogram, which shows it in thickness (Stoker, 1980). The surface can be seen at arthroscopy, and loss of joint cartilage can be inferred on a plain X-ray by noting loss of joint space. This X-ray must be weight-bearing. Cartilage tends to be thicker on the area where the bones bear directly on each other, and less thick where the menisci intervene.

On the tibia it naturally covers the medial and lateral plateaux; it extends over the posterior edge of the lateral plateau to allow the meniscus to slide back in full flexion (3.1). It is not found on the midline strip where the cruciates and the horns of the menisci are attached (3.2). The outer part of the tibial spines is coated with hyaline cartilage, the inner part not (3.3).

The edge of the articular cartilage is palpable at the joint line (though indirectly, through the collateral ligaments and capsule). One can feel here for exostoses if suspecting severe wear or osteo-arthritis.

3.1

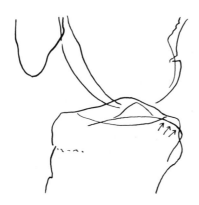

3.2

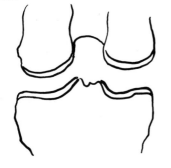

3.3

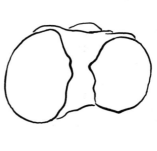

Femoral surfaces

On the femur the areas for the tibia and for the tibio-meniscal articulation are joined to form a large area of articular cartilage (3.5). The edges of this are available to the examining finger, especially in flexion. There is no cartilage on the intercondylar notch of the femur. It is extra-synovial, being where the cruciates attach.

Patellar surfaces

On the patella, the cartilage is in facets as shown (3.4), being essentially flexor and extensor areas for medical and lateral femoral condyles. The small, vertical, medial facet visible here is the odd facet, an interesting structure that is considered on pages 36 & 38.

The articular cartilage of the patella can be directly palpated, which is unusual in joints. See page 41, para 5 for method.

3.4

3.5

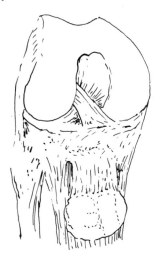

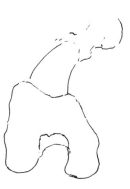

four **The menisci**

General description

The two semilunar cartilages are similar in shape, but there are subtle differences that reflect the movements of the two halves of the joint. Each is crescent-shaped, tethered by an anterior and a posterior horn, and wedge-shaped in section. See (4.1), (4.2), (4.3), and trace of arthrogram (4.4 and 4.5).

Their structure is fibrocartilage, the collagen being arranged mainly parallel to the circumference. This explains why most tears follow that line.

They have various attachments which may be summarised as follows. Their peripheral parts are attached to the capsule, and by that to the femur above and the tibia below. See (4.1) and arthrogram. Their horns hold them to the sagittal centre part of the tibial plateau (4.6). The lateral meniscus also has its own little ligamentous slings that hold it to the intercondylar notch of the femur, as well as being attached to the tendon of popliteus muscle.

Their substance has a slow metabolic turnover, poor repair capability, and only the periphery of an adult meniscus is vascular or innervated. A small inner tear may be painless, though not if it causes locking. The supplies come in to the periphery from the capsule, to which the menisci are attached either strongly or weakly.

4.1

4.2

4.3

4.4

4.5

4.6

4.7

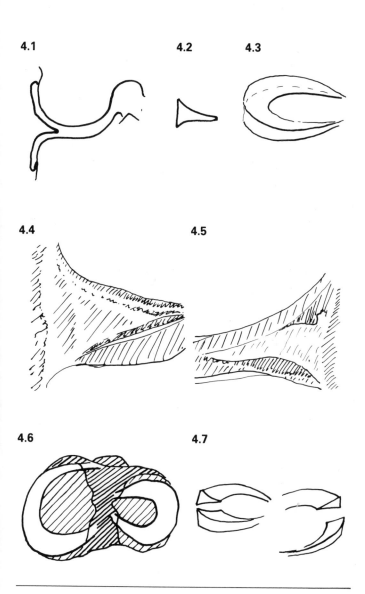

Specific morphology

The difference between the medial and the lateral meniscus will now be discussed under the headings: Shape, Attachment of morns, Attachment to capsule, Attachment by ligamentous slings, and Attachment to tendon. Where possible, structure will be linked with function.

Shape and cross-section

The lateral meniscus is a nearly closed 'C', wide, and thick in section (4.7). The medial meniscus is an open 'C', fairly thin in section, narrow in front and wide behind. The different sections can be linked to the different surfaces of the tibial plateaux and the femoral condyles: especially to the lesser hollowing of the lateral tibial plateau; see (4.8). Now look at the X-ray tracing (4.9) and try to pencil-in where the menisci are.

Functional consequences: From their shapes, both are able to change from a long narrow 'C' to a flat wide 'C', as is shown, exaggerated, in (4.10). Though held centrally, both can move forward and back across the plateau, shown schematically in (4.11).

4.8

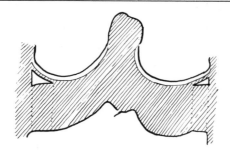

4.9

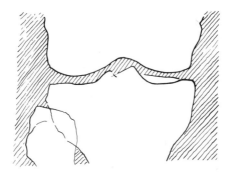

4.10   **4.11**

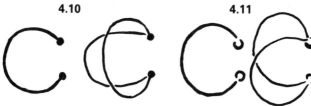

Attachments of horns

The horns of the lateral meniscus are inserted just fore and aft of the lateral tibial spine (4.14). The medial horns are widely separated along the sagittal midpart of the plateau. The horns of the lateral meniscus, being attached so close together, must act almost as a single anchor. They must allow more movement than the medial horns. The two lateral horns may be likened to a single staple holding down a ring—the motion that the staple allows the ring is in an *arc* (4.12).

Functional consequences: A really close look at the surface of the lateral tibial plateau shows how its structure is adapted to movement *around* the lateral spine (de Peretti et al, 1983); see (4.15) and (4.16). Here a small femoral contact area moves across the surface in an *arc*. The medial surface is different; see (4.17) and (4.18). Here a larger femoral contact area remains nearly stationary in the oval hollow. The femoral condyle glides back and forth in the hollow on the medial side. On the lateral side, as it glides, it also rolls across the surface, supported by a meniscus moving in an arc.

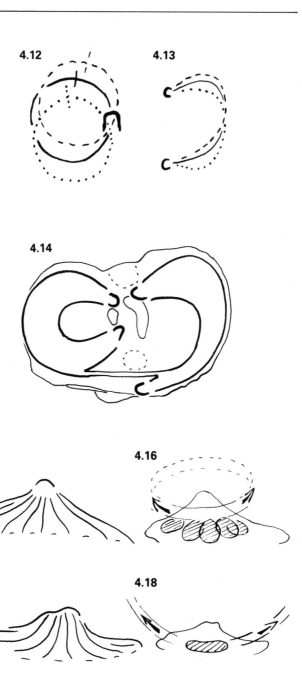

4.12

4.13

4.14

4.15

4.16

4.17

4.18

Attachments to capsule

The periphery of each meniscus is attached to the deep layer of the capsule. On the medial side, the naming of this capsule best follows Slocum & Larson's paper (1968); see theoretical sketch (4.19) and Slocum & Larson's paper, page 212. Here only note that the upper part of the deep capsule, named the medial menisco-femoral ligament, is strong, while the lower part (part of the coronary ligament) is lax. The medial meniscus is thus strongly held to the femur, but loosely held to the tibia. This enables the femur to glide on the tibia for flexion-extension whilst allowing the meniscus to slide over the tibial plateau in axial rotation. The close anatomical relationship of the medial meniscus to the medial ligament is reflected in clinical experience, for example, O'Donoghue's Unhappy Triad, page 106 (O'Donoghue, 1950).

On the lateral side, the same named capsular attachments exist. But they are more lax and attach more distally on the tibia than on the medial side (Stoker, 1980). The lateral collateral ligament is effectively far away, being an extra-capsular structure.

Functional consequences. The capsular attachments are appropriate to a greater amount of movement by the lateral meniscus. O'Donoghue's Unhappy Triad points to the existence of close connections between the medial ligament and capsule and the medial meniscus.

Attachments by ligamentous slings

The posterior horn of the lateral meniscus has two (variable) ligamentous slings (4.20). They pass medially, attaching at the insertion patch of the posterior cruciate ligament, that is, on the inside of the medial femoral condyle (4.21). They divide around the posterior cruciate ligament, one in front (the anterior menisco-femoral ligament) the other behind (the posterior menisco-femoral ligament). The anterior one is the ligament of Humphrey, the posterior one is the ligament of Wrisberg. One or the other may be absent, or both. See Kaplan (1956), which is about the naming of these ligaments, and Last (1948), page 686.

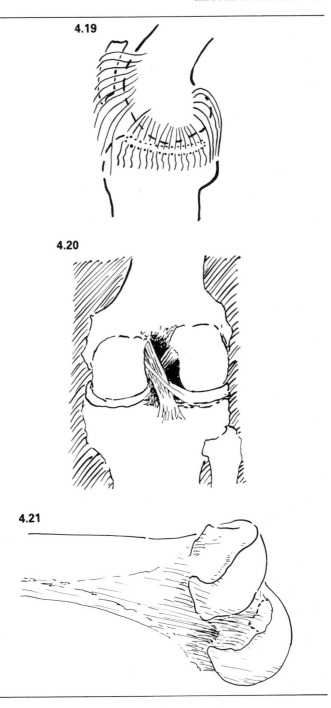

4.19

4.20

4.21

The posterior cruciate insertion patch is eccentric with respect to the axis of the medial femoral condyle (Girgis et al, 1975, p. 221, drawing p. 218). As the joint moves towards extreme flexion, the posterior cruciate becomes tensed (4.22). So also must the anterior and posterior menisco-femoral ligaments become tensed, exerting a posterior and medial pull on the posterior horn of the lateral meniscus. The little ligaments thus help to move the lateral meniscus backwards and medially in the extremes of flexion.

A close look at the lateral tibial plateau reveals a steeply sloping surface at the very back of the plateau, arrowed in the drawings (4.23) and (4.24). That surface is for the lateral meniscus in full flexion (Last, 1948).

A fibrous band joins the front parts of the two menisci; see (4.25) and (4.14). This is called the transverse ligament. In the first drawing, part of the anterior cruciate ligament is seen attaching to the anterior horn of the lateral meniscus (Girgis et al (1975) The cruciate ligaments of the knee joint, p. 218, drawing p. 221). These two anterior attachments become tense at the approach to extension, the anterior cruciate by a similar mechanism (4.22) to that which affects the posterior cruciate in flexion, and the transverse ligament because the medial femoral condyle moves backwards with its meniscus at that stage of movement. Hence there is an antero-medial pull on the anterior part of the lateral meniscus as extension is approached. There is a special part of the lateral tibial plateau, visible on the dry bone, shaded in (4.26), to accommodate this move of the meniscus. It was described in Barnett (1953) Locking at the knee joint, page 93, and figure 3.

Functional consequences: The mobility of the lateral meniscus is caused by and controlled by ligaments. Ligaments pull it backwards in flexion, and ligaments pull it forwards in extension (4.27). The angle of their pull will encourage movement in an arc.

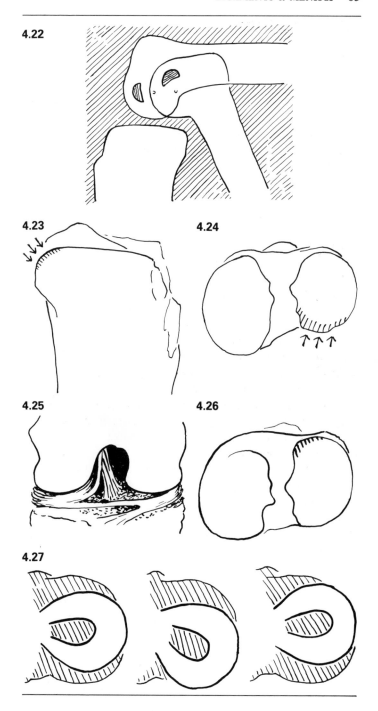

4.22

4.23

4.24

4.25

4.26

4.27

Attachment by tendon: popliteus muscle

The lateral meniscus can also be pulled on by part of the tendon of popliteus muscle, a small muscle that arises from the back of the tibia; see (4.28). The main tendon of popliteus passes under a thickening of the posterior capsule called the arcuate complex, thus entering the joint. It grooves the back of the lateral tibial condyle, and the lateral meniscus; it also grooves the lateral condyle of the femur (in a flexed position), passes deep to the lateral ligament, and attaches to bone near the epicondyle of the lateral femoral condyle (4.29). A small tendon from it attaches directly to the back of the lateral meniscus (4.28). See also Last (1950).

Popliteus actively causes lateral rotation of the femur on the tibia. This can also be called medial rotation of the tibia under the femur. This movement occurs at the very beginning of flexion, and also to a lesser degree throughout the range of flexion (Trent et al, 1976, p. 264). It is said that the slip from popliteus ensures that if the lateral femoral condyle is retracted, the back of the lateral meniscus is as well (Last, 1948, on p. 688, and compare Barnett & Richardson, 1953).

There is an extension of the synovial cavity deep to the popliteus tendons and deep to the proximal part of its muscle belly—compare the lubrication of the tendon of the long head of biceps brachii. This deep pocket or bursa is a site where loose bodies may finish up (4.31).

Functional consequences: As mentioned above, described by Last (1948).

4.28

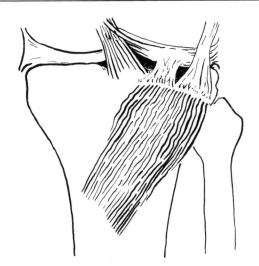

4.29

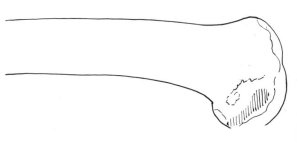

4.30

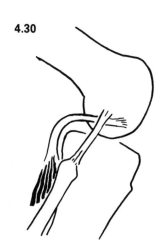

4.31

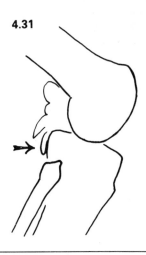

Summary: meniscal attachments

The medial meniscus has firm and extensive capsular attachments to its periphery, and its horns have widely separated insertions on the tibial plateau (4.32). Its capacity for movement is limited.

The lateral meniscus has lax capsular connections, and its horns are attached close together. Considerable movement is possible. Tiny ligamentous slings hold it to specific parts on the intercondylar notch of the femur. They are able passively to move the meniscus, such movement being appropriate for the travel of the femoral contact patch across the lateral tibial plateau.

Summary: the menisci and movements of the knee joint

Flexion-extension: Any pure hinge movement of flexion-extension occurs between the femoral condyles and the upper surfaces of the menisci—shown schematically in (4.33). However, in flexion the lateral meniscus is carried backwards, even on to the steep posterior slope of the lateral tibial plateau (4.34 and 4.37); it returns as the knee returns towards extension. In the last 20 degrees of extension the medial condyle of the femur medially rotates, carrying the medial meniscus back a little, while the lateral meniscus slides forward on to its special extensor area (4.34 and 4.38). These meniscal movements fit with the conjunct rotation that occurs at the knee during flexion-extension.

But in addition, the contact area on the femur for extension is less sharply curved than that for flexion—see the lateral profile of a femur on a lateral X-ray. So as extension is approached, the menisci become squashed out—elongated in an A–P direction. In extension, the contact patch is larger, and longer A–P; in flexion it is smaller, and wider from side to side. See sketches (4.37) and (4.38). See also Walker & Hajek (1972) The load-bearing area in the knee joint.

Rotations. In axial rotation the menisci 'stay with' the femur, and their lower surfaces move over the tibial plateau.

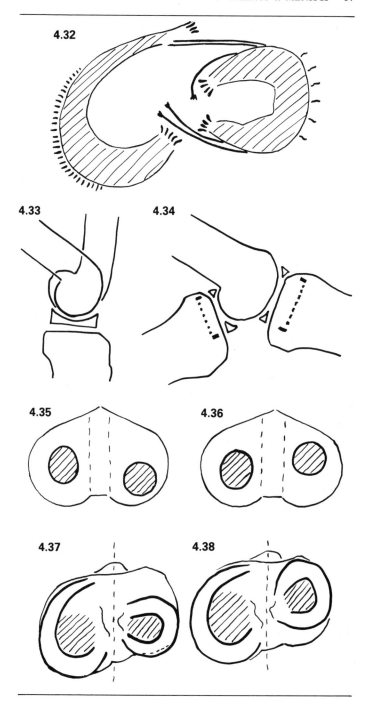

Summary: the menisci and knee function

It is generally agreed that it damages a joint to remove a meniscus. 'Menisectomy is not wholly innocuous'—a quote from Fairbank (1948) Knee joint changes after menisectomy. But it is not generally agreed what they actually do, though there are many ideas. See also MacConaill (1932).

(i) They enlarge the contact area present while a relatively small tibio-femoral contact patch moves across the joint surface. This especially helps the range of flexion.

(ii) They allow two sorts of movement to occur while at the same enlarging the contact areas. (Such dual movement is usually only possible in joints with lax capsules such as ball-and-socket or saddle joints; the latter has a very small contact area, and the former requires great muscle power to control and stabilise movement during weight-bearing.)

(iii) They thus increase the area through which weight is transferred or over which sheer stresses act (Seedhom, 1976).

(iv) They help the lubrication and nutrition of the articular cartilage by sweeping fresh synovial fluid across the joint surface.

(v) They act as load-bearing ligaments, holding the femoral condyles to prevent lateral slide. There is no lateral drawer sign in a normal knee.

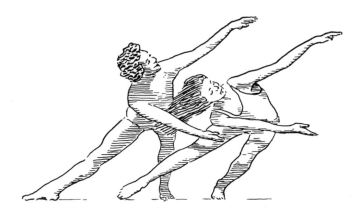

Jonathan Lunn and Lauren Potter, London Contemporary Dance Theatre. (Adapted from photograph by Anthony Crickmay.)

Summary: meniscal dysfunction and the knee

The usual reason for meniscal injuries is asking too much of the knee, mostly in the course of contact sports. Injury to the medial compartment is more common because external force is more common: see (4.39). Such a force opens up the medial compartment of the knee. The medial ligament can become stretched or ruptured, and the strong capsular menisco-femoral ligament may become detached or torn—a peripheral meniscal tear.

The usual signs of chronic meniscal damage are locking or giving way. A persistent effusion may also signal trouble in the joint.

The congenital discoid meniscus is an anomaly found almost always on the lateral side, occurring about once in eighty knees. It may be symptomless, and even if found, it may be left alone rather than taken out. It may cause a snap or a clunk, but the usual reason for discovering one is that it has developed a cyst which presents in the lateral joint line. See Smillie (1948).

The examination of the joint for damage to menisci is covered in the section on Clinical tests for ligaments and menisci.

4.39

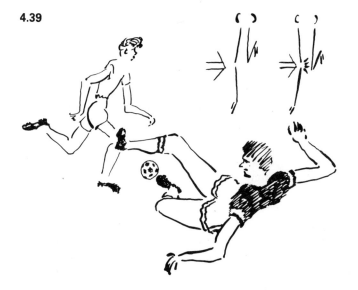

five **Synovium**

Description of tissue

Synovium is a mesothelium, one of the tissues that lines body cavities. Synovium, peritoneum, pericardium and pleura are all mesothelia. (A factor that induces a synovial effusion may also cause effects in the other mesothelia too.) Each is a very thin layer of cells (5.1), called the serous layer (S), on a fibrous tissue backing, called the fibrous layer (F). The cells produce synovial fluid. There is a sensory nerve supply in the underlying fibrous layer.

Location of synovium

As in all joints, the synovium of the knee completely lines the inside of the fibrous capsule and is attached to each bone at the edge of the articular cartilage. The actual line of attachment is usually beyond the edge of the joint surface, a pocket being left to allow for movement. Synovium does not cover the bearing surfaces of the joint, so it is not found on the articular cartilage or on menisci; see (5.2). Synovium conceals the cruciates from the arthroscope. It covers the fat pads that fill the odd nooks and crannies of the joint, such as the one deep to the ligamentum patellae. It also forms fringes of finger-like processes (villi) that extend into the joint (5.3). Both fat pads and villi can be injured by getting pinched, giving pain (Hoffa, 1904). This pain can be found by deep palpation either side of the patella or patellar tendon, in the joint line. The synovial folds or plicae are covered later, p. 76.

5.1

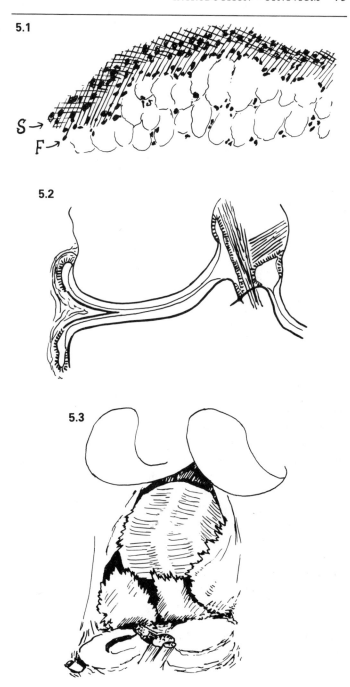

S→

F→

5.2

5.3

Synovial cavity

The synovial cavity has a medial compartment, a lateral compartment and a patellar compartment, and they are connected. The medial and lateral compartments are there because there is a nearly complete median septum that divides the joint in the sagittal plane. The appearance is as if the cruciates have invaginated the synovial cavity from behind (5.4). The cruciates are thus extra-synovial, but intra-capsular. (An anterior cruciate tear will bleed and produce a haemarthrosis; a posterior cruciate tear will also bleed, but as the posterior capsule is usually also torn, the blood dissipates in the calf, giving no haemarthrosis but posterior bruising.) The two halves of the cavity are connected anteriorly, between the anterior cruciate and the infra-patellar fat pad. The arthroscope gets access to the joint through incisions either side of the infra-patellar fat pad.

The cavity extends over the edges of the tibial and femoral joint surfaces at the joint margins. See (5.5). It also extends out as pockets under tendons that are intimately involved with the joint, for instance the popliteus bursa and the medial gastrocnemius bursa. The bursae are considered later.

The cavity continues up around the patella, forming the para-patellar recesses (5.6). They lubricate the side attachments of the patella. They become visible when swollen by a joint effusion. The cavity extends proximally for two or three fingers' breadth above the upper pole of the patella as the supra-patellar bursa. This is really the ventral capsule folded up in extension; see (5.7) and (5.8). There is an equivalent pouch formed by the posterior capsule in flexion.

The medial para-patellar recess is a preferred site for synovial needle biopsy. The supra-patellar pouch is the usual site of puncture when drawing fluid off the knee. It is also a good place to palpate when looking for the thickened synovium (pannus) of rheumatoid arthritis.

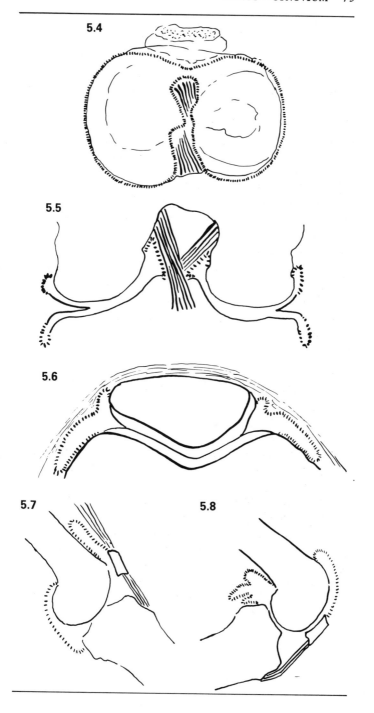

5.4

5.5

5.6

5.7   5.8

Synovial plicae

A plica is a fold of synovium that protrudes inwards. Surgeons that use arthroscopy can visualise a plica that is causing pain in the knee. See Glasgow et al (1981).

The superior plica is probably an embryological remnant, being the remains of the division between the supra-patellar pouch and the knee joint proper (5.9). There may be an almost complete transverse fold, a finger's-breadth above the upper pole of the patella. More usual is a crescentic remnant on the medial aspect. For review, see Pipkin (1971).

The medial plica is a vertical fold of synovium found along the medial patello-femoral joint line, or just behind (5.9). It intrudes into the medial para-patellar pouch, and may injure the cartilage locally. There may even be bony changes, visible on X-ray. Tenderness, with or without a palpable band, may be elicited over the antero-medial femoral condyle. Unlike the one above, this plica may be derived from scar tissue, from repeated blows to the medial aspect of the joint—sporting injuries!

Bursae round the knee

There are many bursae around the knee joint. Some are connected to the joint cavity, and some are not.

Anteriorly: the sketch (5.10) shows (a) the supra-patellar bursa, mentioned above, being the ventral capsule folded up in extension; (b) the pre-patellar bursa overlying the kneecap, a subcutaneous bursa of use when crawling, laying carpets, scrubbing floors etc., hence 'house-maid's knee'; (c) the deep infra-patellar bursa, for lubricating the patellar tendon on the tibia in extremes of flexion; and (d) the superficial infra-patellar bursa, which lubricates the movement of skin over the tibial tuberosity, and is in use when kneeling, hence 'clergyman's knee'. The supra-patellar bursa is connected to the knee joint, the other three are not.

5.9

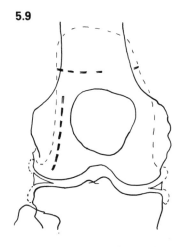

5.10

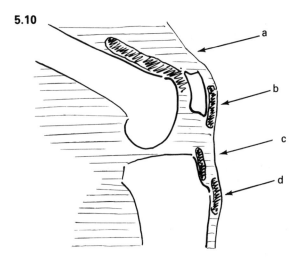

Laterally, there are two bursae that help sliding between tissue planes; see (5.11). One is between the lateral ligament and the tendon of popliteus, just below the lateral epicondyle (b). The other is between the lateral ligament and the inserting tendon of biceps femoris; it is just above the fibular styloid (d). Neither of these connects to the joint cavity. There is also a lateral gastrocnemius bursa (a) and a popliteus bursa (c), serving obvious functions deep to their tendons as shown. The first is sometimes, and the second is always, connected to the joint cavity.

On the medial side (5.12) there is a gastrocnemius bursa which always connects to the joint (a); an extensive semi-membranosus bursa, between the tendon and the back of the tibia, and the tendon and the medial head of gastrocnemius (b)—this also connects to the joint. There is also a series of bursae that lie both deep and superficial to the medial collateral ligament (Brantigan & Voshell 1943). The one underlying the pes anserinus (tendons of sartorius, gracilis and semitendinosus) is shown here (c). Also shown are two that are related to the medial ligament (d) and (e). None of these connects with the joint cavity.

5.11

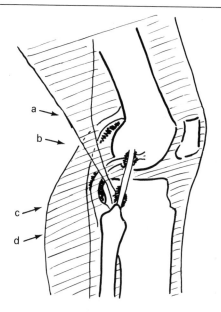

5.12

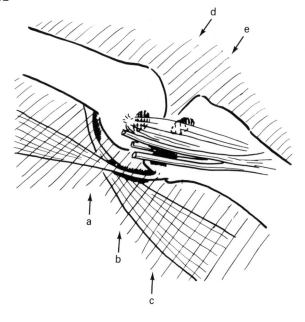

Cystic swellings about the knee

Any cystic swelling around the knee, suspected of being a bursa, may have one especial characteristic: if it is connected to the joint cavity, it should be soft in flexion but become tense and hard in extension. This is because extension is the close-packed state of the joint, when the volume inside the joint is least.

A popliteal cyst is a cystic swelling behind the knee—the name is not specific. It may be an enlarged semi-membranosus bursa, or it may be a simple herniation of the synovium through the posterior capsule. The simple herniation is said always to be secondary to something that is causing a persistent synovial effusion in the joint.

Synovium—structure and function

Apart from providing lubrication, synovial fluid contains nutrition for the articular cartilage; see the diagram (5.18). From where it is secreted at the periphery of the joint, it has to be conveyed to all the articular cartilage. This happens incidentally as the joint movements sweep the fluid across the articular surfaces. Fat pads press against the surface that is not articulating, and deliver fluid directly on to the joint surface (5.15, 5.16, 5.17) and synovial villi deliver deeply between the joint surfaces. The joint movements then carry this fresh fluid away to more distant areas of the articular cartilage.

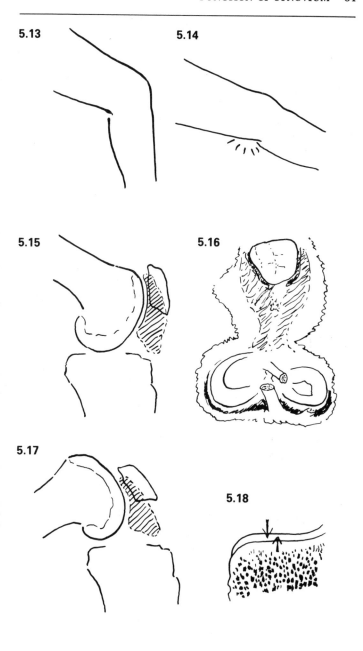

The surface layer of the articular cartilage is supplied by diffusion, but deeper layers are reached by fluid that is squeezed out and then drawn in by the elastic recoil. This occurs just as it does in a sponge, during intermittent loading. (The deepest layer gets nutrition from the subchondral bone.) Thus to care for cartilage, a joint needs regular swept movements and on-off loading, throughout its range (5.19). See Radin & Paul (1972).

Synovium—dysfunction: effusions

Effusions (*i*). If a knee is sprained (*definition*: partial tears in ligament or capsule), the synovium takes part in the general inflammatory reaction. The resulting synovial exudate becomes a joint effusion. When there is a joint effusion, that fluid in the joint has not got the normal ability to lubricate and feed the articular cartilage. Exercising on a joint with an effusion damages its articular cartilage.

Effusions (*ii*). Detecting an effusion by patellar tap: the supra-patellar pouch is squeezed by the upper hand, and the lower hand presses the patella sharply against the femur (5.20). The patella is felt to hit the femur with a clunk if the test is positive. The test can be negative with a large effusion, for the capsule can be so tense that the patella cannot be depressed. Nor will it reveal a small effusion; the next test is for that.

Effusions (*iii*). The cross-fluctuance test: with the joint in extension, the fluid is milked upward out of the medial para-patellar pouch, and then out of the supra-patellar pouch downwards and laterally. See (5.21). Keeping the supra-patellar pouch flat, the free hand compresses the lateral para-patellar pouch, pushing any fluid present medially. The fluid may be seen to bulge out the skin medially; see (5.22). See also Stickland (1984) p. 146.

Effusions (*iv*). If there is a lot of fluid and the capsule is tense, the knee will not be able to attain the position of close-pack, where the intra-synovial volume should be least. It is usually held slightly flexed, and cannot be fully extended. Such a knee will often yield over 100 ml fluid on aspiration, whereas normal synovial volume is 5 ml or less.

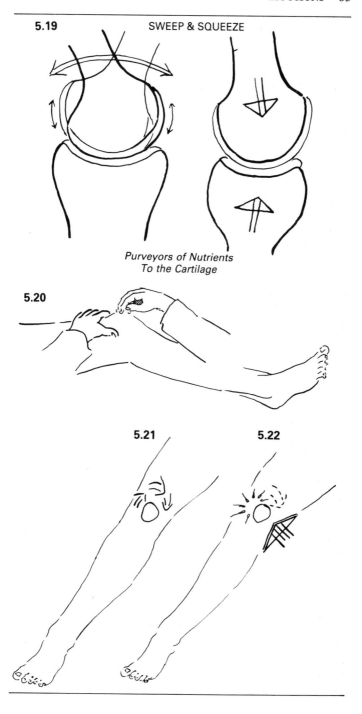

5.19 SWEEP & SQUEEZE

*Purveyors of Nutrients
To the Cartilage*

5.20

5.21   **5.22**

Effusions (v). A really tense effusion is usually accompanied by painful muscle spasm. This is because the stretching of the capsule causes enormous numbers of proprioceptive stretch-receptors to fire off, with consequent reflex contraction of large numbers of muscle fibres. If the effusion is bloody, the irritation of the synovium will cause pain and even more reflex muscle spasm. Such a joint cannot properly be examined, hence the need to aspirate and then examine, often under anaesthetic.

Effusions (vi). Aspiration of a tense effusion will relieve pain; a bandage must be applied immediately to prevent recurrence. Full asepsis must be observed. The safest entry point is into the lateral side of the supra-patellar pouch, below vastus lateralis. A medial entry here would have to pass through vastus medialis, and below the patella one would encounter the infra-patellar fat pads and might injure the infra-patellar nerves to the joint. See the diagram (5.23).

Access to synovium: to palpate synovium to check for thickening, the supra-patellar pouch is generally chosen. Quadriceps must be relaxed. Sometimes the edge of the synovium can be 'rolled' beneath the fingers.

5.23

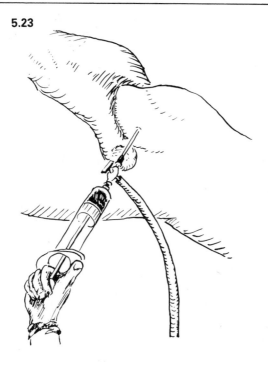

six Fibrous capsule and ligaments

General structure

The fibrous capsule of the knee is made of collagen-elastin, with a network of blood vessels and nerves. The collagen gives strength, especially if thickened to form capsular ligaments. The blood vessels care for the metabolic needs of the tissues; they bleed if there is a sprain, but multiply to form granulation tissue in the subsequent repair process. The nerve endings are chiefly of mechano-receptor type, for joint proprioception, but there are also pain receptors and tendon organs. For joint neurology see Wyke (1967).

At its simplest, the capsule can be merely a fibrous backing for the synovium, looking like a thin transparent membrane. But in the knee, parts of it are thickened, forming parallel strands of dense, glistening collagen that are ligaments. Although ligaments are often drawn in diagrams as separate entities, looking like flexible cast-iron pillars, their fibres shade into the fibres of the nearby capsule, and their edges have to be cut by the dissector who defines them.

Ligaments do 'bind one bone to another'. But in a complex mechanical joint like the knee, they provide flexible checks that ensure that a movement proceeds smoothly, as if along a controlled path. They provide the boundaries of the path—compare fairground gondola in diagram (6.1). See also Struben (1982)—a fascinating, short paper.

6.1

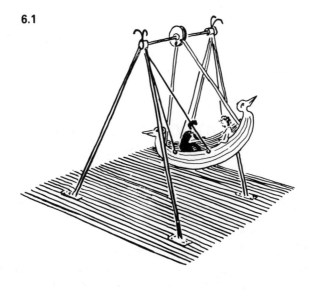

The ligaments of the patella

As the quadriceps pulls on the patella, its transverse stability is ensured by a sheet of collagenous material either side. This is called the patellar retinaculum. In dissection it appears as layer after layer of fibres, vertical fibres from the quadriceps interleaved with different oblique fibres between patella and femur.

It prevents excessive side-to-side movement of the patella in its groove. In full extension, the patella is out of the groove and the retinaculum is loose enough to allow the patella to be lifted for palpation of the margins of the articular cartilage (Fig. 2.32). The medial patellar retinaculum is one of the factors helping to prevent lateral dislocation of the patella; see patella, page 46. Contrariwise, repeated lateral dislocation may be treated surgically by cutting the (tight) lateral patellar retinaculum—a 'lateral release'.

Introduction to capsular and extracapsular ligaments

This introductory section exists only to explain the general arrangement and nomenclature of the ligaments. Like any other overview presented to help understanding, it will be inaccurate in some specifics.

The capsule is in several layers, with thickenings in it termed capsular ligaments. These thickenings may only be present in one part of that layer of the capsule, according to the need for stabilising influences.

The deepest layer is just outside the synovium. At the sides it joins the menisci to the two knee bones (6.2). The upper part of this is called the menisco-femoral ligament. It is only well developed on the medial side (i.e. the lateral side is too mobile). The lower part of it is called the coronary ligament. (*Corona* is a Latin root meaning 'around', or all round.) It is present on both sides. See (6.3).

6.2

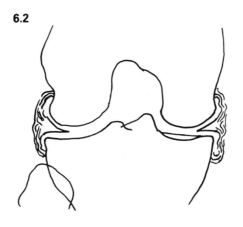

6.3

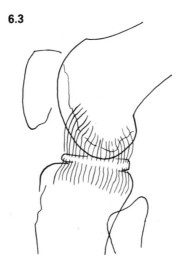

The next layer contains the major capsular ligaments of the knee. The patellar retinaculum is part of this layer too. Medially is the medial ligament proper, or tibial collateral ligament. It extends back to the postero-medial capsule. See schematic diagram (6.4). Sometimes both parts are together described as the medial ligament, or medial complex. Posteriorly, the thickenings are called the oblique popliteal ligament (which is the knee's posterior ligament), and the arcuate ligament, which is partly a capsular guard over the penetrating popliteus tendon. Next is the postero-lateral complex. In some writings this may include the arcuate complex and the lateral collateral ligament. Capsular thickenings appear to be weak in the lateral and antero-lateral quadrant, probably because of the strength of the overlying extra-capsular ligaments.

Superficial to the capsule are the extra-capsular ligaments. They are the lateral ligament proper, or fibular collateral ligament, and the iliotibial tract. See (6.4) again.

6.4

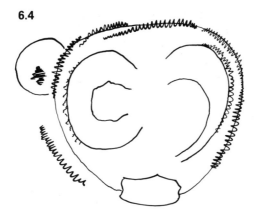

seven The lateral and postero-lateral ligaments

Introduction

In this area there is variation between individual knees, variation between different papers and books, and variation in nomenclature. Apart from standard books and some dissections, papers found useful were the following:

— Seebacher et al 1982 The structure of the postero-lateral aspect of the knee.
— Hughston et al 1976 Classification of knee joint instabilities, Part 2: The lateral compartment.
— Last 1948 Some anatomical details of the knee joint.

The deepest layer of the capsule is that part that connects the meniscus to the femur above and the tibia below. The lower part is called the coronary ligament. The upper part, though present, is weak, and seems not to have a name. (On the medial side it is called the medial menisco-femoral ligament.) The coronary ligament is strong but lax, allowing for axial rotation, which occurs at the knee joint at the tibiomeniscal interface. The inner layer becomes thickened postero-laterally to form part of the arcuate complex. That is briefly described in the next layer, but more fully with the posterior capsule.

Outside the capsule proper is the lateral collateral ligament, or fibular collateral ligament. A capsular leaf overlies it, which thickens up behind to form the fabello-fibular ligament (Seebacher et al, 1982), the short external ligament of old terminology (Last, 1948).

7.1

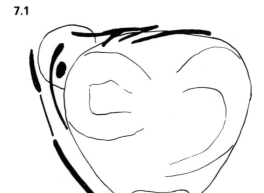

The lateral ligament

The lateral ligament is a cleanly rounded ligament, roughly the size of half a pencil. Above, it is attached to the epicondyle of the lateral femoral condyle; below, to the styloid process of the fibula (7.2). The tendon of biceps enfolds its lower end, and can be a guide to it. In extension it angles back as it passes distally. In flexion it angles forward, for the lateral femoral condyle moves to the back of the tibial plateau in flexion; see (7.3). To palpate your right lateral ligament when sitting, contract sartorius and rest the right lateral malleolus on the left supra-patellar bursa; then allow the right knee to relax and drop. The taut cord is easily felt.

The lateral ligament is fairly constant. But the reinforcing structures behind the lateral femoral condyle from the fabello-fibular ligament, the arcuate complex and the lateral end of the oblique popliteal ligament, are variable.

The lateral complex is assessed clinically by the varus stress test, page 146. Postero-lateral weakness combined with anterior cruciate insufficiency is detected by the history, and by the pivot shift test, page 160.

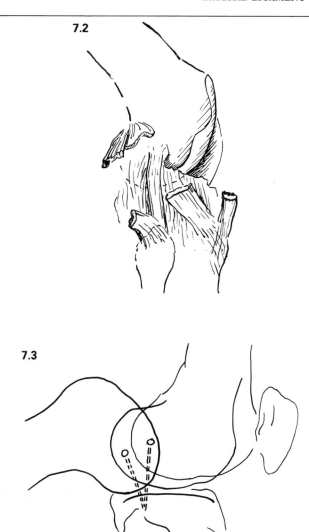

7.2

7.3

The fabello-fibular ligament and arcuate complex

The fabello-fibular ligament is a broad thickening that passes downwards and forwards to the fibula from behind the lateral femoral condyle (7.4). A leaf from it overlies the lateral ligament and attaches to the capsule in front.

The arcuate complex must be described here, though it is part of the inner layer; see (7.5). It originates as part of the deepest layer of the capsule, being an arched thickening over the penetrating tendons of popliteus muscle. Laterally it attaches to the postero-lateral tibia and to the fibula.

Function

The three ligaments all stabilise the lateral compartment of the knee, though it is hard to say exactly when or how. The fibular collateral ligament, for example, is actually lax, *loose*, throughout flexion, only becoming tight near full extension (Brantigan & Voshell, 1941). That ligament is however expressly angled to resist the terminal movement of conjunct rotation.

The iliotibial tract

Outside all these ligaments is the iliotibial tract, together with the strong fascia derived from biceps tendon (7.4). The tract has never been proved to have a stabilising function at the knee, though this may just be because no experimental work has been done, and that in turn because the tract is not commonly a clinical problem. We should note, however, that its direction and strength is similar to the medial ligament; also that the underlying capsule seems to have no need for strengthened capsular elements. It is known as a 'dynamic stabiliser' of the knee. This means that it is believed to contribute to knee stability during walking and running, but no-one has ever proved it by experiment. In the end, its function may be revealed when too much of it is taken for fascial repair material, for reconstructing the anterior cruciate ligaments of expensive football players, for example!

Its function in posture has been described in a *most* interesting paper; see Evans (1979)!

7.4

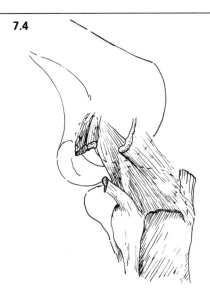

7.5

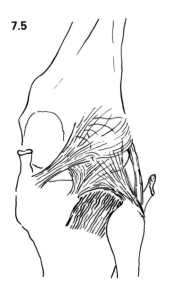

eight The medial complex

The finest way to learn about this area is by doing dissections, but the following papers will also be found useful, for they combine gross anatomy with mechanical experiments and clinical experience. Slocum & Larson (1968) 'Rotatory instability of the knee' is full of anatomy correlated with clinical findings. Warren & Girgis (1974) 'The prime static stabiliser of the medial side of the knee' is more specific and numerate, but corroberates Slocum generally. Brantigan & Voshell (1941) is also a fine paper which links structure and function in the joint, especially contrasting the medial compartment with the lateral compartment.

Deep layer

It is again useful to see this complex as a deep layer and a superficial layer, both capsular. The entire upper origin is centred around the medial epicondyle of the femur.

The deep layer is strongly attached to the medial meniscus. The upper half holds the meniscus to the femur, and is the medial menisco-femoral ligament. The lower half attaches distally just beyond the articular margin, and is the coronary ligament (8.1). Though they are both thickened, the coronary ligament is lax enough to allow the meniscus to move over the tibia in axial rotation.

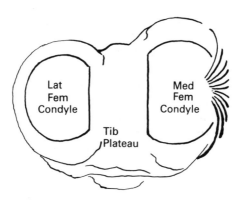

Lat
Fem
Condyle

Med
Fem
Condyle

Tib
Plateau

8.1

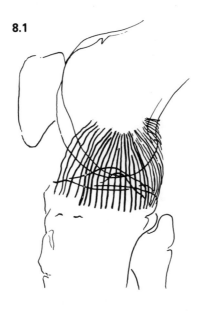

Superficial layer

Outside the deepest layer, but still part of the capsule, is the medial complex. The names are rather variable here, but whatever the names are, there is a middle one-third and a posterior one-third, see (8.2). These may together be called the medial complex or the medial ligament. Or the middle one-third might be called the medial ligament proper, while the posterior one-third be called the oblique part of the medial ligament, or the postero-medial complex. The anterior one-third is just known as the antero-medial capsule.

The medial ligament occupies the middle third of the joint line; see (8.2). Above, it is attached around the medial femoral epicondyle, i.e. near the axis of hinge movement in flexion. At the joint line it cannot be separated from the deeper capsule and the periphery of the medial meniscus. Below the joint line, a deeper part attaches to the tibial condyle, while the strong parallel fibres of the superficial part angle forwards to attach distally a full hand's breadth below the joint line. Here it lies beneath the inserting tendons of the pes anserinus—sartorius, gracilis and semi-tendinosus. See (8.2) again.

Bursae are often found in this region, especially where soft tissue planes rub over each other or pass over protuberances.

The postero-medial complex or oblique part of the medial ligament is found on the side and back of the medial femoral condyle.

8.2

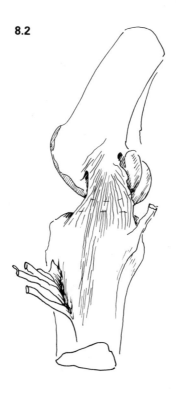

Tension in the medial complex

First of all, a note on degrees of tension: in this book, a ligament that has no tension in it is either lax, loose, or slack. One that has some tension in it is called tight or tense. One that is taking a lot of tension is called taut.

Tension of the medial ligament in different arcs of flexion. In the close-packed position of full extension, the medial femoral condyle is thrust backwards (tightening up the postero-medial complex), and the medial femoral epicondyle lifts away from the tibial plateau, tensing the medial ligament proper. See (8.3). Thus in close-pack, almost all the ligament is taut. In the early ranges of flexion, the medial ligament proper remains tight, but by 15° of flexion the whole medial condyle has moved forward towards the centre of the plateau, so that the postero-medial complex becomes much less tense. See (8.5). As flexion continues, it is the front and the middle parts of the medial ligament proper that remain tensed; see (8.6). The postero-medial complex is now slack. By 80° of flexion, the middle part of the medial ligament remains tense, but its anterior and posterior parts are lax. See (8.7).

Note that through the working range of the joint the greater part of the ligament proper remains tense—which is appropriate. But note also that different parts of the ligament are tense at different degrees of flexion. So joint strains (tears of those parts that were tense and maintaining stability) will occur in different parts of the ligament according to the position of the joint at the time of the injury. In this way a really accurate history can be a guide for the examining finger, thus enabling diagnosis and treatment to be very specific.

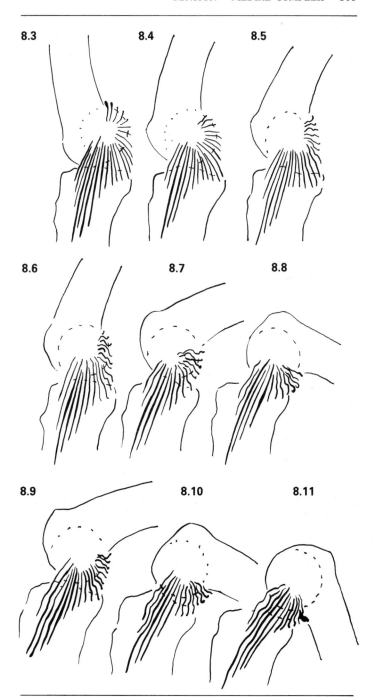

Movements of the medial ligament. In the later degrees of flexion, the medial ligament slides posteriorly across the edge of the tibial condyle, moving forwards again in extension. See (8.12) which is traced from Brantigan and Voshell, page 49. This is the sort of movement that requires a bursa, and a fairly constant one lies deep to the anterior edge of the ligament here.

Function of the medial complex

(i) It resists valgus (abduction) strains. It is helped in this by the anterior cruciate ligament. A moderate valgus strain will sprain the medial ligament. A strong stress will tear the medial ligament and strain or lengthen the anterior cruciate; see (8.13). A huge stress will rupture the medial ligament and the anterior cruciate, and possibly the posterior cruciate too. The clinical test for this sort of injury is the valgus stress test, which is described and rationalised in the section on ligament tests.

(ii) It resists external rotation of the knee (see Slocum & Larson, 1968, p. 213 et seq.; Warren & Girgis, 1974, pp. 670 & 671). The sequence of injury from an external tibial rotation force is: first, rupture of the medial collateral ligament, and then rupture of the anterior cruciate. The clinical tests for these injuries are: (a) the range of external tibial rotation, usually measured at 80° or 90° flexion; (b) the rotatory instability test of Slocum et al (1976), on pages 64 and 65 of his paper and page 154 here; and (c) the external rotation recurvatum test, which is similar to (b) but in full extension. These three are also described and explained in the section on ligament tests.

(iii) It helps the anterior cruciate ligament to resist anterior glide of the tibia beneath the femur. See (8.14). The clinical use of this is that an anterior drawer (normal or abnormal) of tibia beneath femur should be abolished by external rotation of the tibia.

See also 'Clinical tests for ligament function' at the end of this book.

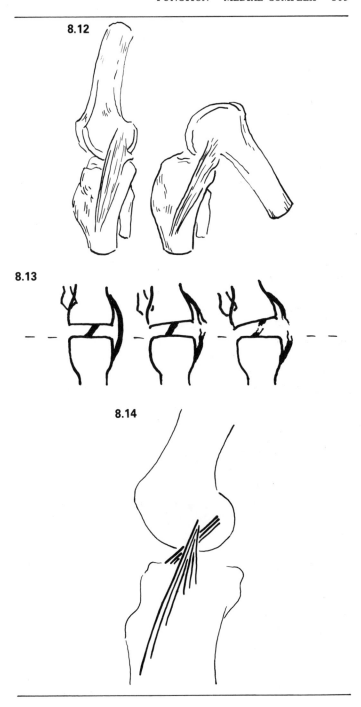

8.12

8.13

8.14

(iv) It contributes to the close-packed condition. If you see the outline of the femoral condyles as a wheel-and-a-wedge, the epicondyle is in the centre of the wheel, and that is the upper attachment of the medial complex. As extension is approached, the epicondyle begins to lift off the tibial plateau (see (8.15)) as the wedge wedges. Hence at extension the whole medial complex becomes stretched. It thus resists hyper-extension and contributes to the close-packed state. The effect of terminal hyper-extension with its conjunct rotation, on all the ligaments, is considered at the end of this section under 'The close-packed condition,' page 125.

(v) Its length is functional. In the final 15° of extension, the medial femoral condyle moves backwards (8.16) as the terminal conjunct rotation 'locks' the joint. The femoral condyle must be on a long rein to allow this excursion. The long rein is the medial ligament. The bursa beneath the ligament allows it to slide over the deeper structures. (On the lateral side the long rein is the iliotibial tract and the *laxity* of the lateral collateral ligament.)

The medial ligament is closely related anatomically to the medial meniscus, and functionally to the anterior cruciate. An injury which turns up with depressing frequency is a combination of torn medial ligament plus torn anterior cruciate plus torn medial meniscus. This is known as 'O'Donoghue's Unhappy Triad', after a paper by that author; see O'Donoghue, (1950).

The medial complex is assessed clinically as follows. (i) Lateral angulation is tested by the valgus stress test, page 142. (ii) Prevention of a normal or abnormal anterior drawer test by external tibial rotation is the basis of Slocum's rotatory instability test, page 154. (iii) The prevention of anterior glide of the medial tibial condyle only is described by Trickey (1982).

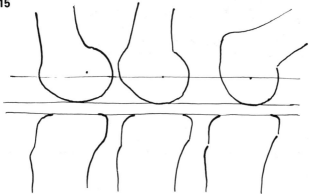

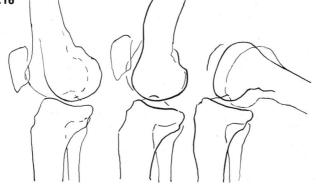

nine The cruciate ligaments

General

These two ligaments occupy the intercondylar notch; they are named from their tibial attachments. They are extra-synovial (diagram 5.5), i.e. they cannot be inspected at arthroscopy unless the synovium is cut or breached. They are strong, having a breaking strain of about 60 kg (Trent et al, 1976, p. 270), and about as thick as a pencil. Older cruciates tear with less strain, younger ligaments being some three times stronger (Noyes & Grood, 1976). Their primary role is to control antero-posterior movement, but they also have a marked effect on varus-valgus resistance and on the resistance to rotation.

The literature on the cruciates is extensive, especially if you include arthroscopy and the various repair procedures. The four papers cited here are chosen because they are primarily antomical and also very clinical. They are also very fine papers.

—Brantigan O C, Voshell A F (1941) Mechanics of the ligaments and menisci of the knee joint.
—Girgis Fakhry et al (1975) The cruciate ligaments of the
knee joint.
—Trent P S et al (1976) Ligament length patterns, strength,
and rotational axes in the knee joint.
—Markolf K L et al (1976) Stiffness and laxity of the knee—
the contribution of the supporting structures.

9.1

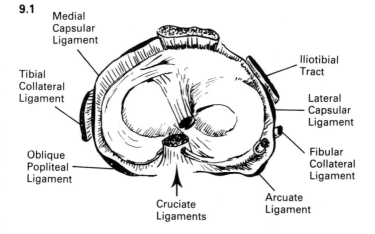

Medial
Capsular
Ligament

Iliotibial
Tract

Tibial
Collateral
Ligament

Lateral
Capsular
Ligament

Oblique
Popliteal
Ligament

Fibular
Collateral
Ligament

Cruciate
Ligaments

Arcuate
Ligament

Anterior cruciate ligament (9.2)

Position and structure

The tibial attachment is quite forward on the tibial condyle, though not far off being central (9.1, 9.2, 9.3). It overlaps the attachment area of the anterior horn of the lateral cartilage; here slips from it pass to this horn.

From there the ligament passes backwards, laterally, and upwards; it attaches to the lateral condyle of the femur way back in the inter-condylar notch (9.4).

The attachment on the femur is specific (everything about this joint is specific, for its biomechanics to happen, but more is known about the anterior cruciate ligament than other structures). It is a half-moon, nearly in line with the femoral shaft, and it is placed just posterior to the transverse axis of flexion-in-flexion (9.5). Note that relative to the axis of hinge movement in extension, it is well posterior and distal. So in theory it should remain fairly constant in length (and thus in tension) in the flexor range from about 60° to 120°, but become progressively stretched from about 60° down to extension.

The collagen fibres of this ligament are arranged somewhat in a spiral manner, an arrangement commonly seen in Nature where great forces are involved, e.g. tree trunks. Being composed of collagen-elastin, and of average length 21 mm, each ligament can only lengthen by some 8% before rupture, i.e. by 1.7 mm.

The anterior cruciate is extrasynovial, see (5.2) and (5.4). Hence it is difficult to visualise well through the arthroscope unless the synovium is torn or slit open. But it is within the fibrous capsule of the joint, so that blood from a torn ligament produces a haemarthrosis. Compare posterior cruciate, page 116.

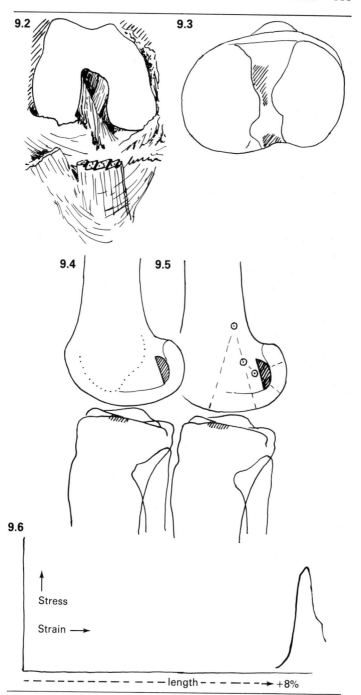

9.2

9.3

9.4

9.5

9.6

Stress

Strain →

← – – – – – – – – – – length – – – – – – → +8%

Movements

In flexion (9.8), the ligament becomes twisted (X-shaped) so that only the antero-medial band remains taut (Girgis et al, 1975, p. 229; Slocum & Larson, (1968), p. 214), say about a quarter of the ligament. As the joint moves from flexion towards extension (9.9), two things happen. First, the ligament untwists as the attachment turns, and its fibres become nearly parallel. Second, the two ends of the ligament get pulled apart, as the femoral insertion patch gets forced further off the tibial plateau. This effect is mechanical, caused by the spiral or wheel-and-wedge shape of the femoral condyle. See (9.7) and (9.9) here, and page 33. At extension, further extension cannot happen unless the ligament 'gives'. See also the mechanics of 'close-pack' at the end of the section on ligaments, p. 124.

In extension, the anterior cruciate occupies a small antero-lateral notch of its own in the main intercondylar notch of the femur (9.10). This little notch can be seen on some intercondylar views on X-ray. In anthropological circles this notch affords evidence that the knee extended fully, and thus that posture was erect. Neanderthal man had no notches. His gait is thus supposed to have been crouching, not upright. Australopithicus has the notch.

9.7

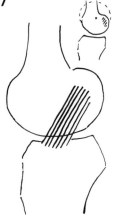

9.8

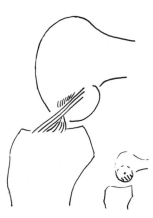

9.9

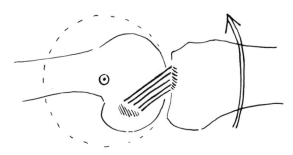

9.10

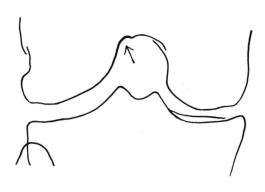

Functional and clinical

Just by looking at the direction taken by the anterior cruciate ligament, and with some idea of what it looks like from the side, from in front, and from above, one can see that it can:
—resist forward movement of the tibia under the femur (9.11).
—resist lateral rotation of the femur on the tibia (9.12). See Trent et al, page 266.
—resist varus/valgus forces, in conjunction with the collateral ligaments (9.13).

Knowledge of these mechanical functions is implicit in the correct performance of the clinical tests for a suspected cruciate injury. Ligament tests are described and explained on page 138 et seq.

The specific tests for the anterior cruciate ligament are the anterior drawer tests, page 148, and the pivot shift test, page 160. The recurvatum test and the valgus or varus stress tests could detect anterior cruciate tears when other ligaments are also involved.

Tears of the anterior cruciate can occur with surprisingly small force, especially if rotation stresses were suffered. Internal tibial rotation can tear the ligament by causing excessive lengthening, theoretically by more than 1.7 mm; see paragraph above in 'structure' and (9.14) & (9.15) here. External tibial rotation actually slackens the anterior cruciate, and is moreover strongly resisted by the medial collateral ligament. But in contact sports it is often combined with a substantial valgus strain. This combined strain ruptures first the medial collateral ligament, then the anterior cruciate ligament; see (9.16). This is the beginning of O'Donoghue's Unhappy Triad (O'Donoghue, 1950).

A forced hyper-extension injury will also stretch this ligament (9.17) but since almost all the ligaments are taut in this position, the anterior cruciate damage will be part of a multiple ligamentous injury.

If a haemarthrosis is suspected clinically, then a major ligament tear must also be suspected. Torn anterior cruciate should especially be eliminated.

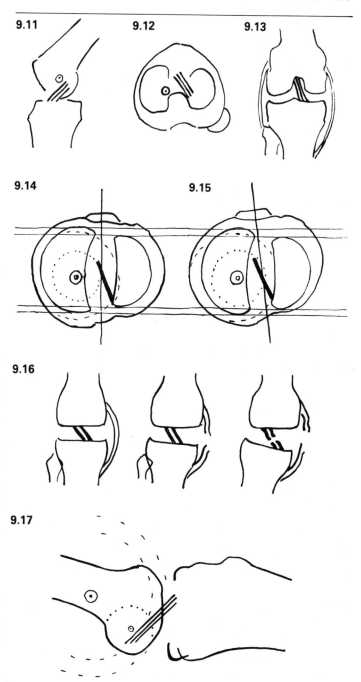

9.11

9.12

9.13

9.14

9.15

9.16

9.17

Posterior cruciate ligament

Position

Its tibial attachment is way back on the posterior edge of the tibia, extending some way down the posterior aspect of the bone (9.18 and 9.20). It is more on the back than on the top of the tibia. From here it passes anteriorly and upwards, just medial to the anterior cruciate, and attaches to the medial femoral condyle.

Like the anterior cruciate, its femoral attachment is placed most specifically with respect to the axis of rotation-in-flexion (9.19). The shape is again of a half-moon, but the flat is horizontal. The flat is again placed right next to the axis of hinge movement in flexion.

Like the anterior cruciate, the posterior cruciate is extra-synovial. A bleed from a torn posterior cruciate is unlikely to produce a haemarthrosis, however, because the posterior capsule is usually torn as well, and the blood escapes into the calf. Compare anterior cruciate, page 110. The circumferences of both calves should be measured if a posterior cruciate tear is suspected acutely.

Movements

If the position of the posterior cruciate is projected on to the shape of the tibial plateau, the ligament is seen to overlie the average centre of axial rotation; see (9.21). Hence the frequent clinical statement that the axis of rotation of the knee is the posterior cruciate ligament.

It is instructive to make a tracing or cut-out of the lateral view of the femur with the posterior cruciate patch marked on it, and move it over a lateral outline of the tibia. In this way the movements of the femoral insertion patch are shown here (9.22). It appears that in the working range of the joint—20° to 30°—the posterior cruciate is least stretched. In extension, the patch becomes lifted away from the tibial origin as the epicondyle lifts. This must stretch the ligament. As flexion proceeds, the femoral insertion patch is seen to rotate over the top of the axis of hinge movement in flexion. The ligament must be getting considerably tensed as this happens.

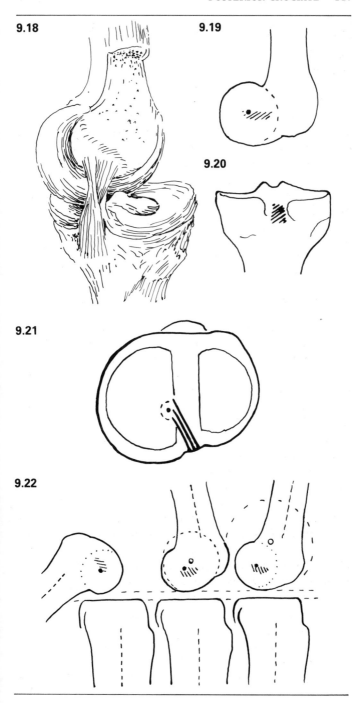

9.18

9.19

9.20

9.21

9.22

These simple mechanical deductions (9.23) are broadly confirmed in the paper by Trent et al (1976), the graph on his page 267 showing the rising tension in the posterior cruciate as flexion proceeds. He has the lowest tension at 15°, the tension rising from there towards either flexion or extension.

Near extension, only a small part of the posterior cruciate is taut (9.27). This is the posterior part, going to the posterior end of the femoral attachment (Girgis et al, 1975, p. 244 & Fig. 16). This posterior oblique band remains on stretch from extension through early flexion, when the 'big circle' part of the femoral surface is bearing. But as flexion proceeds it relaxes (9.25), and the rest of the ligament tightens up. The spin of the femoral condyles takes the insertion of the main part of the ligament up over the axis. So the majority of the ligament becomes tensed as flexion proceeds.

Functional and clinical

It helps to prevent the tibia from moving backwards underneath the femur, for example when landing from a height. Injury of this type is exemplified by the dash-board injury— a direct blow to the front of the upper tibia in a passenger seated with knee flexed (9.28).

It helps all the other ligaments to resist further extension at terminal extension—close-pack. A hyper-extension force strong enough to do damage may tear both cruciates and the medial collateral ligament.

The posterior cruciate ligament is assessed clinically by the posterior drawer test, page 158. It is not easy to do well, but most of all it is not easy to remember to do at all. Posterior cruciate damage is often found months after a severe road accident (9.28), where at first other things were more important. The posterior cruciate can also get torn when a knee is forcibly abducted or adducted in extreme flexion, when the ligament is already at full stretch (9.23).

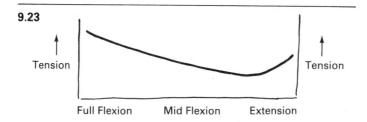

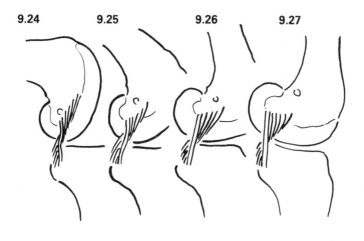

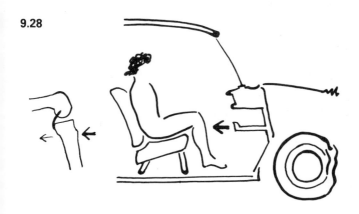

It is often said to be the 'fundamental stabiliser of the knee' (e.g. Hughston et al, 1976, p. 160) because it seems to be near the axial centre of rotation. This centre of axial rotation changes with flexion and extension (Trent et al, 1976), and is perhaps best thought of as being sited between the arcs of action of the ligaments that are taut. In the usual working range of the knee—20° to 40°—this means the medial collateral ligament and the two cruciates; see (9.29) here. It moves closer to the posterior cruciate in flexion because the posterior cruciate becomes tight then, but moves forward in extension as the anterior cruciate tightens up. In the last few degrees of extension it moves laterally, because the lateral ligament tightens up in extension, (9.30) and (1.17).

Underneath a pile of bodies at some friendly sporting occasion, a player may find his knee subjected to an irresistable rotation stress while it is buckled up beneath him. This can rupture the posterior cruciate. Such a rupture may not produce a haemarthrosis (see above), but should be suspected if extensive bruising of the calf develops.

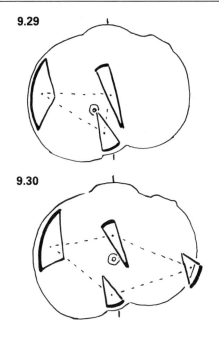

9.29

9.30

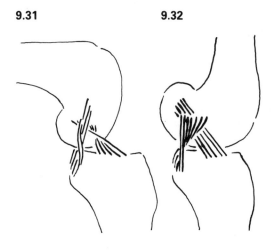

9.31

9.32

ten Stability from ligaments

It is still true to say that anterior-posterior stability is chiefly achieved by the cruciates, though a positive anterior drawer test usually means medial ligament damage also (10.1).

It is also still true to say that the collaterals bear the burden of varus-valgus strain. But clinically a severe valgus strain will tear first the medial complex, and then a cruciate ligament (10.3 and 10.4).

As for rotary strain (10.5 and 10.6) it is generally accepted that external tibial rotation is chiefly controlled by the medial ligament (Slocum & Larson 1968; Warren & Girgis, 1974), and internal tibial rotation by the anterior cruciate (Trickey, 1982; Stickland, 1984). These are clinical judgements as well as experimental. Anyone in the field of trauma or sport (same thing really) would stress the contribution of good muscles to compensate for knee instability.

When someone has a knee that is unstable due to lax ligaments, they often complain of uneasiness or giving-way when *turning*. It is as if muscle build-up cannot compensate for rotary instability. Hence the knee brace found most useful by these unfortunates is a de-rotation brace.

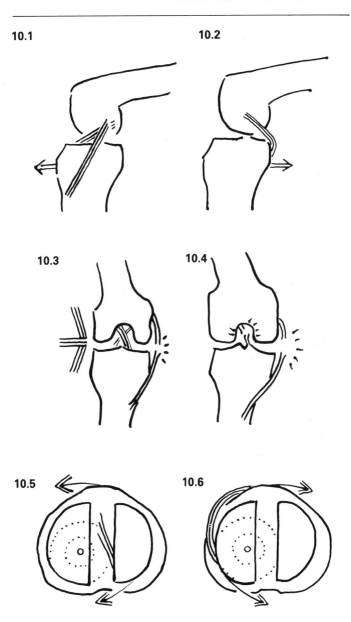

eleven Close-pack and loose-pack

Throughout the working range of flexion, only a part of each ligament is taut. Their elasticity is easily overcome, so that clinically we find a degree of natural laxity in flexion. It is normal to find 10–20° of laxity in rotation or in varus-valgus tests in flexion, and some anterior drawer. This working range is known as Loose-pack, a term first coined by MacConaill in the 1930s.

But as extension is approached, all ligaments slowly become stretched. The reasons are: (i) the lifting of the femoral epicondyle off the tibial plateau by the spiral or wheel-and-wedge effect; this lifts the proximal attachments of both cruciates and both collaterals away from their tibial attachments; see (11.1) and (11.2); (ii) the accelerating conjunct movement of medial femoral rotation; this especially affects the three peripheral ligaments—the medial, the lateral, and the oblique popliteal; see the diagram (11.3).

As the joint goes through this stage, the elasticity of the ligaments is taken up, and the joint surfaces become increasingly thrust together. Small movements, e.g. by menisci (Barnett, 1953), allow further limited movement, but then the relentless stretching continues.

With further stretching, the collagen passes through its elastic phase to its non-elastic phase. The ligaments then resist further stretching, so that no more extension is possible.

At this point there is a balance of powers: extensor force equals resistance to stretch of ligaments plus resistance to deformation of joint surfaces and subchondral bone. Less extensor force, and the elasticity of the collagen springs the joint out of extension. More extensor force, and ligament collagen begins to tear (a sprain). See Smith (1956).

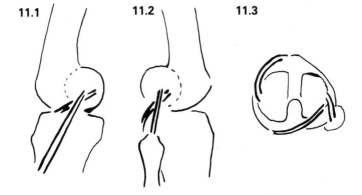

11.1   11.2   11.3

When this balance is reached, the tightness of the capsular ligaments squashes any synovial pouches, so that the intra-synovial volume is very small. Lastly, the joint is so constructed that at this stage the bearing surfaces are most closely fitting and have the largest area in contact.

This stage is known as the 'close-packed condition of the joint' (MacConaill, 1964, page 363). In this state we nowadays say that:

— most ligaments are maximally stretched
— the intra-synovial volume is least
— the articular surfaces are maximally congruent
— the articular surfaces are strongly apposed.

The close-packed condition is used by the body (Evans, 1985), and is useful to anyone who has to examine joints.

Day-to-day uses of a close-packed knee

In the ordinary 'stand-at-ease' position, the knee is nearly straight, but is not closely packed. But if the person leans back on one leg in the asymmetrical standing position (Smith, 1953), then the knee does extend into close-pack. In this position it is nearly immovable. Synovial joints are usually thought of in terms of movement, yet here is the knee exhibiting the opposite state, namely, not mobility but stability.

The stability is ensured because the body's centre of gravity passes in front of the transverse axis of the joint in this position, holding it extended into close-pack, and thus 'locked'. The hip is also similarly held in extension because the line of the body weight passes behind it, holding it in extension too. The knee also has an additional factor, for the iliotibial tract holds the knee into extension as well, having been tensed by the relaxed adduction of the hip (Evans, 1979). The result is the posture of relaxed standing known to us all. See (11.4).

11.4

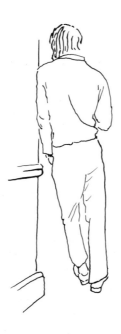

Clinical uses of close-pack

Because the ligaments are taut, and the joint surfaces both most congruent and thrust together, this position is a position of great stability. It stands in contrast to the rest of the range, which can be called loose-pack, where play in the joint is detectable clinically and where stability is substantially aided by muscles.

But close-pack is stressful for a joint, for the ligaments are under stretch, and the articular cartilage and sub-chondral bone are compressed. However, a stressful state is useful in Medicine: for instance a sugar tolerance test can give information about the state of the islet cells of the pancreas, and an exercise ECG can test heart muscle and its blood supply. So to put a joint into close-pack will ask a question of the ligaments, the articular surfaces and the subchondral bone, as well as of the intra-synovial volume. The question is, 'Are you all right?'

If a joint can painlessly achieve a normal close-pack, there cannot be a lot wrong with it. So this can be used as a quick test to exclude pathology, just as the physiotherapist uses her 'quadrants'. Or else it can be used to find the joint that is giving trouble, for example in a child with a limp who cannot give a history anyway.

Abnormal states of close-pack can also be useful, namely the recurvatum test and its variants; see page 170.

Inability to achieve a close-packed knee is seen when there is a large joint effusion, and when a bucket-handle tear is impinging between the medial femoral condyle and the front of the medial tibial spine as extension is approached. See opposite. It is also common in old age, for whatever reason.

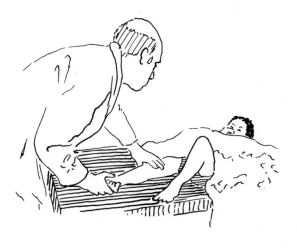

twelve Stability of the joint

Muscular factors

The hamstrings and the quadriceps are the two main muscle groups of the knee, but the hamstrings are primarily hip muscles, for their EMGs indicate that they function with the glutei as anti-gravity hip muscles. Thus the quadriceps group are the most important muscles of the knee joint.

The stability of the knee, like any other joint, is shared between muscles, ligaments and articular surfaces; see (12.1). Instability due to ligamentous laxity can be overcome by increasing the power of the muscles to compensate (12.2). Thus most ligamentous injuries are given quadriceps exercises which will alleviate symptoms provided that the injury is not severe. Quadriceps exercises can also help other forms of knee injury, so they are frequently used as a cure-all.

In the absence of systemic disease or neurological reasons, wasting of the quadriceps is a symptom of trouble in the knee. Wasting may be due to pain inhibition, whether from the bone in osteo-arthritis or the capsule in inflammation or effusion. It may be due to disuse as when a patient unconsciously 'spares' a joint that is unstable. Or wasting may be due to the loss of local reflex arcs, such as reduced afferent impulses due to tearing or incision of capsular mechano-receptors, or altered proprioception due to laxity in the capsular structures. The negative afferent impulses from pain or the reduced afferent impulses from proprioceptive loss will then have their effect on the motor neurones to the quadriceps. Any reduction in the mechano-receptor afferent barrage will reduce the normal recruitment of motor neurones that occurs, especially at the beginning of a movements; see (12.4). Since recurrent knee sprains or a major tear cause substantial loss of proprioceptive end-organs in the capsule, with some

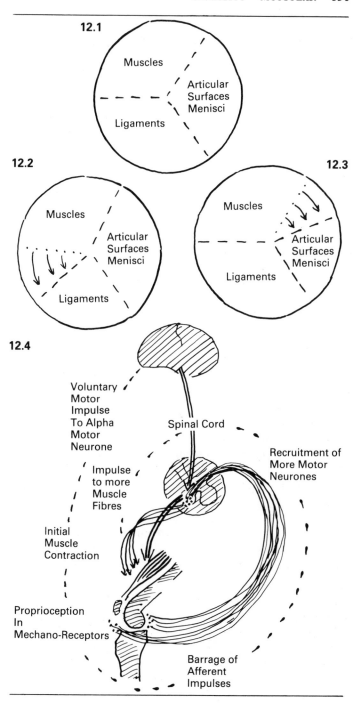

injuries no amount of work can make quadriceps regain its former bulk.

Osgood–Schlatter's disease

Active children in their teens may present with a painful anterior tibial tuberosity. It is clinically tender, and may be swollen, and X-rays may show partial avulsion of the tuberosity (12.5 and 12.6). This is an apophysitis called Osgood–Schlatter's disease. The pain may keep a child off strenuous activity for years.

Stability of the joint— neurological factors

The joint capsule is richly supplied with proprioceptive end-organs, the majority of which are mechano-receptors; see the review by Wyke (1972).

There are capsular mechano-receptors that are low-threshold and fast-adapting; these signal 'my tension has been changed'. There are also those that are low-threshold and slow-adapting; these signal 'my part of the capsule is under tension'. Essentially the first signals movement and the second one signals position. There are also high-threshold mechano-receptors, called Golgi tendon organs, chiefly in the major ligaments. Their impulses are inhibitory to the motor neurones— these are interesting clinically, see later. Pain impulses are also inhibitory.

The afferent impulses from the capsular mechano-receptors travel to several places. Amongst other destinations they go to the neurones in the spinal cord, for spinal reflexes to aid voluntary movement; see (12.4). (Note that the patellar tendon reflex is a reflex derived from the muscle spindles in the vasti, and is nothing to do with the neurology of the joint.) The afferent impulses from the joint also go to the the cerebellum, to programme it with joint position, so-called unconscious joint proprioception. These provide the background for extra-pyramidal motor impulses. They also go to the cerebral cortex, for conscious joint position sense. This provides the background for pyramidal (conscious) motor impulses.

12.5   **12.6**

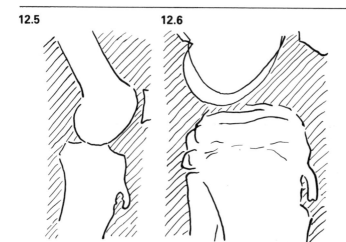

Clinical aspects—anterior knee pain

Pain felt in the front of the knee may be caused by disease in the hip. The characteristic gesture is a rubbing of the front of the distal thigh, with the fingers over the knee-cap. The hip should always be checked if there are knee symptoms, but anterior knee pain especially should alert the examiner.

Pain receptors in the capsule and the subchondral bone are probably responsible for the severe pain felt when a knee 'jams' from an impacted loose body. Pain receptors in the synovium are intensely irritated by a haemarthrosis.

'Giving way'

'Giving way'—a neurological phenomenon: the simplest example of this is when the patient gets up (to to put a kettle on) after prolonged sitting (in front of TV). At the first step the joint collapses, because it has 'gone to sleep'. This is probably due to minimal local ischaemia to nerves, caused by an awkward sitting position which has squashed local capillaries that supply the nerves.

The 'giving way' that happens with chronic meniscal injuries or ligamentous laxity is a reflex phenomenon.

A small piece of dislodged meniscus may suddenly become 'jammed' between the joint surfaces. It deforms the subchondral bone and stretches the capsule. Both of these cause pain. Pain produces inhibitory impulses on the motor neurones at the appropriate spinal level, the muscles switch off and the knee 'gives way'. Here the pain comes before the giving way.

When the ligaments and capsule have been damaged, they are often lax. Normally the joint passes smoothly through its range of movement controlled by ligaments, different parts of which are taut in different positions (12.7). The effect is of moving between firm walls that allow no 'chatter' (side-to-side movement) (12.9).

But if part of a ligament or capsule is lax, the smooth control is lost (12.8), and the femoral condyles can 'bounce' from one ligamentous restraint to the next (12.10). In this way sudden stresses on the capsule are likely to occur.

12.7

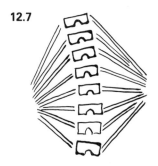

12.8

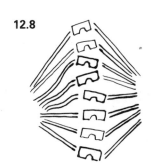

12.9

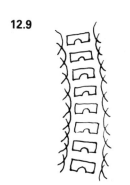

12.10

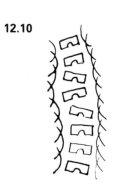

Such a sudden, intense stretch is just the stimulus that fires off the Golgi tendon organs, specialised high-threshold, fast-adapting mechano-receptors that inhabit ligaments and tendons. They are only set off by great stresses, and they are protective.

When fired off, their afferent stimulus acts on the segmental motor neurones, inhibiting nearly all muscular activity at the joint. The knee gives way without warning. This can be quite painless, if a trifle surprising.

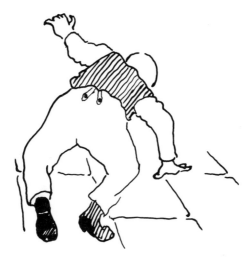

thirteen Clinical tests for ligament and cartilage damage

Examining the acute knee

The tests as described here assume a quiet knee, with little fluid, minimal pain, and no muscle spasm. This may be good for description and for learning, but does not resemble the acutely injured joint.

When an injury is recent, joint laxity is often concealed by swelling, effusion and muscle spasm, and a sensitive examiner may not feel able to examine the joint properly because of pain.

Nevertheless, somebody has to grade the severity of an injury in the acute state, if only to label it as an IDK— Internal Derangement of the Knee (often known as 'I Don't Know'!). Here, good history-taking may be all-important, but a gentle yet firm examination will often confirm the initial suspicions.

The examination of the recently injured knee is similar to that of a painless knee, except that every test has to be done within the small range of painless movement available. It is helpful to realise that a ruptured ligament is not painful to test, because there is nothing to pull on. Indeed a severe and multiple ligament injury may be far less painful to examine than a nasty sprain.

This section seeks primarily to explain in simple terms the mechanical basis of each test. The normal anatomy and mechanics of the ligaments and menisci are covered in earlier sections. Some readers may wish to refer to these, for to understand how a joint expresses its abnormality, one must thoroughly understand the normal.

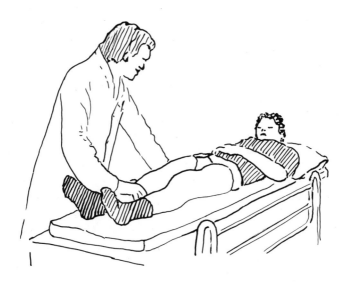

Introduction—mechanical basis of tests

The various tests performed to detect damage to capsule or ligament may appear very different in different hands, but the mechanical principles on which they are based remain the same. They have been described by Hughston et al in their 1976 papers (Hughston et al 1976 Part I and Part II); the paper by Markolf et al (1976) is excellent and full of relevant experimental data.

The pathological anatomy of the ligament tests was described by Trickey (1982). Stickland (1984) contains a description of both the subjective and objective examination of the joint, including the assessment of the ligaments. The tests are also well illustrated in a book, *Clinical Orthopoedic Examination*, by McRae (1983).

In the search for ligament damage the joint is stressed in an attempt to produce movement which should be prevented by ligament or capsule (13.1). As in any other hinge joint, tests are done both for excessive angulation and for excessive glide. Of the angulation tests, there are the varus and valgus stress tests, and the check for excessive extension. The anterior and posterior drawer tests search for excessive glide between the joint surfaces in the sagittal plane. Medial or lateral rotation of the tibia during a drawer test can give added information that can reinforce or complement the primary tests.

Knee ligaments are very strong; it is not uncommon for the inexperienced to miss injuries because insufficient force has been applied. The force needed is not great. What is needed is the knack of applying the force rather than great strength to apply it. No attempt should be made to overcome pain or muscle spasm by force. They should be respected as danger signals. They signal that something is wrong till proved otherwise. Muscle spasm that is painless can conceal joint laxity: it is one cause of a false negative result, particularly in the anterior drawer test.

Each ligament has one primary function and at least one other function. The sketch (13.5) shows the stress primarily resisted by the anterior cruciate, i.e. anterior glide. The sketch (13.6) shows a second function, restraining valgus, and (13.7) another function, restraining axial rotation. Each

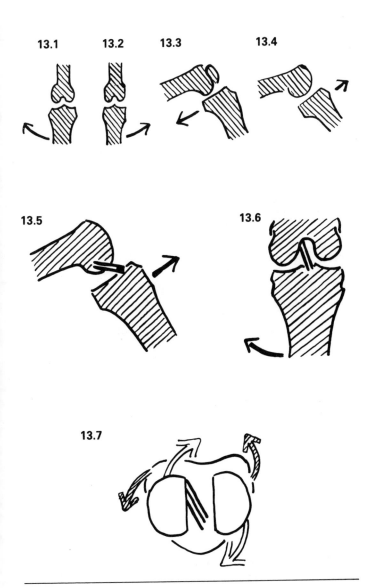

clinical test stresses the joint in one direction. The resistance of that stress is usually the primary task of one ligament and the secondary task of another ligament. See, for example, anterior tibial glide, resisted by the anterior cruciate and medial ligaments (13.8); and valgus stress, resisted by the medial ligament and anterior cruciate ligaments (13.9).

So a severe valgus stress in a sports incident might tear the medial ligament, but only strain the anterior cruciate. Gross stress would tear both. When that patient's knee is tested clinically, a positive valgus test indicates medial collateral damage. A strongly positive test suggests damage to medial structures *and* the anterior cruciate.

Each test thus gives results on one or two ligaments, according to the degree that it is positive; see (13.11) and (13.12). Similarly, one can 'get at' a ligament clinically in two ways, by testing its primary function and also by testing its secondary functions.

The valgus stress test

Principles

The principle here is to try and open up the medial side of the joint by applying an angulating force; see (13.13). The force is an abduction force, i.e. a valgus stress, which may be applied in a variety of ways. See (13.14) here, and (13.19) and (13.20), next page.

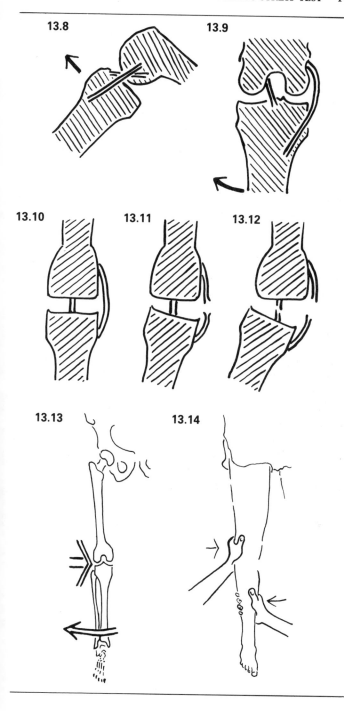

It is self-evident that the medial ligament should resist this force, but it is not so obvious that the cruciate ligaments should also; see (13.15).

This is not a test to be measured by a goniometer, but by hand and eye. Experienced hands often search for the clunk that occurs as the tibia returns to meet the femur, *after* the valgus stress. So they will 'gap' it first as far as possible (13.17), and suddenly return it to neutral (13.18). The appearance may be of just a simple jiggling movement, but it has two parts. During the valgus stress one looks for excessive angulation, either by eye or by actually feeling for gapping in the joint line, (13.20). During the return movement one feels for the clunk.

The test is not initially performed in extension because small increases in medial ligament length (sprains) cannot be detected then. This is because all the other ligaments are tight and help to prevent the angulation, so hiding any deficiency of the medial structures.

Methods

There are many ways of doing this test. Two are sketched here, and should need no further description (13.19 and 13.20).

The valgus stress test is first performed at about 15° to 30° of flexion. Some 'give' is normal at this angle; it should gradually diminish to nothing as extension is reached. Excessive 'give' is judged by experience, as well as by comparison with the other side. If abnormal laxity is found at 15° to 30° flexion, the test would be repeated in extension.

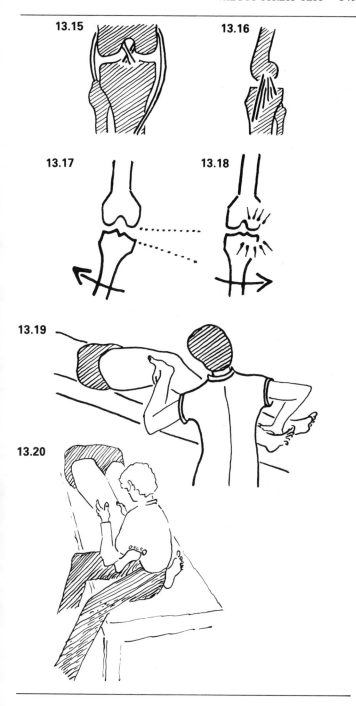

13.15

13.16

13.17

13.18

13.19

13.20

Results

A positive valgus stress test indicates damage to medial structures, including the medial ligament (13.22). A strongly positive test indicates additional damage to structures in the sagittal midline of the joint, such as the anterior cruciate ligament (13.23). If the test was grossly positive, there could be damage to both the cruciates and the posterior capsule, as well as to the medial structures.

If the valgus stress test is at all positive in full extension, when all the ligaments should be taut and resisting any movement, this indicates considerable damage to midline structures as well as medial structures. ('When moderate or marked relaxation is present—on valgus strain in extension—the lesion will usually be found to include the posterior cruciate ligament.'—Slocum, 1968, p. 219)

A positive valgus stress test should be conjoined with the results of the rotatory instability test (of Slocum), which is described in the section on the anterior drawer sign, p. 155; that is also a test for the medial structures.

The varus stress test

Principles

Force is applied to produce an adduction angulation at the knee, a varus stress. The methods used are similar to those of the valgus stress test, see previous page. Again, full extension is not the position for first carrying out the test, for the reasons given in the description of the valgus stress test.

As in the valgus stress test also, though a positive result may be seen as excessive angulation, the examiner may first be alerted by the unusually loud clunk as the lateral tibia returns to its femoral counterpart.

Method (13.24)

This is initially performed with the knee joint at about 15° of flexion. Methods are similar to the valgus stress test (13.19).

13.21
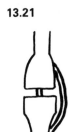

13.22
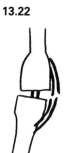

13.23
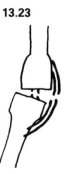

13.24
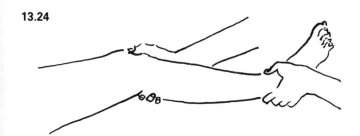

Results

There is normally some 'give', more than on the medial side, but it should diminish sharply to nothing when extension is close. A positive result is gauged by experience and by comparison with the other side. It indicates damage to lateral structures, including the lateral ligament.

If the test is strongly positive, or if it is at all positive in full extension, there could also be damage to midline structures such as cruciates.

The anterior drawer tests

Principles

The anterior cruciate ligament clearly limits forward gliding movement, provided that the test is done in flexion, ie. not in be helped by the medial ligament (13.26), but the angulation of that ligament is less appropriate, and there is more length available for elastic increase in length.

The clinical estimation of this anterior glide is called the anterior drawer test. It is normal to have some anterior drawer movement, provided that the test is done in flexion, ie. not in close-pack. In a normal anterior drawer test, when the tibia is jerked forward, it commonly swivels slightly into external rotation (13.27). This is because there is more anterior cruciate forward length available then (see (13.28) and (13.29)), the centre of rotation being medial to the line of the ligament (data from Trent et al, 1976). Since this normal external rotation component depends on an intact anterior cruciate, a pathological anterior drawer usually lacks this rotary element. The end-feel is also different, and this is explained in Slocum & Larson's 1968 paper, p. 215, top; also on pp. 10 and 11.

13.25

13.26

13.27

13.28

13.29

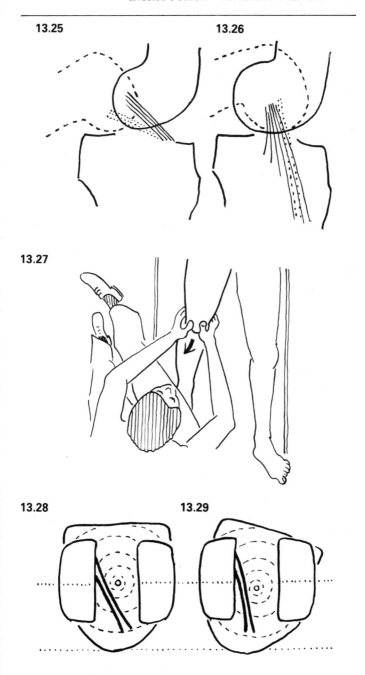

The majority of the anterior cruciate is taut in full extension (13.30) (Furman et al, 1976). But this is closepack, so any small increase in length would be concealed by the tightness of all the other ligaments. One test is thus done just off extension, at 15° flexion, when most of the ligaments have become less taut, see graph (13.32). That is Lachmann's test.

Through most of the flexor range, only a small part of the ligament is tight at any time (13.31). At 80° flexion it is the anteromedial band (Furman et al, 1976). So at 80° the classic anterior drawer test is for the antero-medial band; the 15° Lachmann's test is for the majority of the ligament, that is, the postero-lateral band. With complete rupture they will of course both be positive.

If the anterior drawer is positive in full extension, it must mean damage not only to the anterior cruciate but to other ligaments, especially the medial ligament (with its forward angulation).

Modifications of the anterior drawer test: The normal 'give' of a normal anterior drawer test occurs because there is available elastic increase in length of the ligaments. If by some manoeuvre one ligament can be tightened—'winding up a ligament'—the 'give' may be eliminated.

Thus from a neutral anterior drawer position, a rotation of the tibia externally will tighten up the medial ligament; see (13.33). Hence failure of a normal anterior drawer to be eliminated by external tibial rotation indicates medial laxity. This is the rotatory instability test of Slocum (1968, p. 216). Or a positive anterior drawer sign that is not eliminated by external tibial rotation indicates laxity of the anterior cruciate and medial structures. This is sometimes shortened to 'antero-medial instability'.

On the other hand rotation of the tibia internally tightens up both cruciate ligaments (13.34). So a normal anterior drawer should be eliminated by internal rotation of the tibia. Or a positive anterior drawer (anterior cruciate damage), still present despite internal tibial rotation, suggests posterior cruciate damage also.

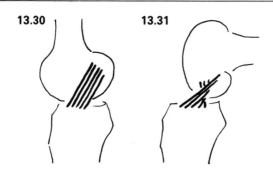

13.30   **13.31**

13.32

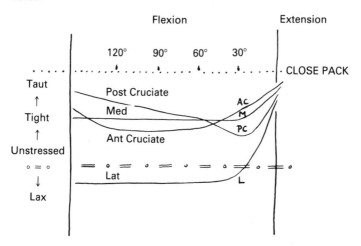

| | Flexion | | | | Extension |
| | 120° | 90° | 60° | 30° | CLOSE PACK |

Taut
↑
Tight
↑
Unstressed
○ = ○
↓
Lax

Post Cruciate

Med

Ant Cruciate

Lat

AC
M
PC

L

13.33   **13.34**

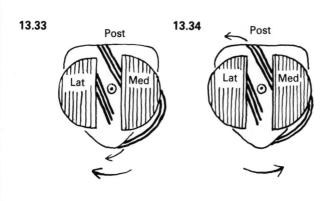

Post   Post

Lat   Med   Lat   Med

Method

The anterior drawer test at 15° of flexion (Lachmann's test) can be done from standing or from sitting. The hands must be placed in the hollows above and below the knee, the upper one laterally, the lower one medially; see the sketches (13.35) and (13.36). Hence when you change legs, you change hands. The tibia is then jerked smartly forwards and backwards in the search for excessive 'play'. It is difficult to do this test on legs that are large, or with hands that are small!

Lachmann's test is especially valuable for joints that are painful, because there is very little disturbance of the knee.

For the ordinary anterior drawer test, the knee is at 80° or so, and is usually stabilised by the examiner sitting on the foot (13.37). The index fingers first ensure that the hamstrings are relaxed—hamstring spasm can mask a positive anterior drawer sign. The tibia is then jerked forward sharply, returned, then jerked again, searching for antero-posterior 'play'.

Results

A positive Lachmann's (15°) test indicates damage to the whole anterior cruciate ligament. A positive 90° test suggests damage to part of the anterior cruciate—the antero-medial band—with or without the rest of the ligament.

A positive result in full extension is a serious sign. It indicates damage to the anterior cruciate ligament plus at least one other ligament, as well as considerable capsular damage.

If a positive result is found, the other knee must also be tested and possibly the thumbs and the elbows as well, in case all the joints are naturally lax (see p. 7). Hence a positive anterior drawer is a matter of comparison as well as of experience. It would be unwise to define a positive result in centimetres.

A positive anterior drawer and a positive posterior drawer each appear as excessive antero-posterior laxity; it is important not to get them muddled up.

13.35

13.36

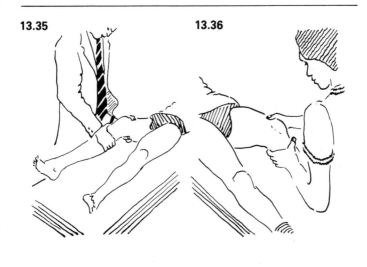

13.37

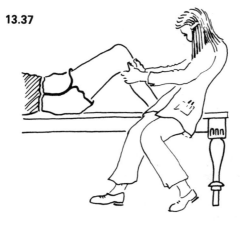

The rotatory instability test of Slocum (Slocum & Larson, 1968)

Principles

See principles of the anterior drawer tests, page 148, briefly summarised thus. With the knee in the anterior drawer position, external rotation of the tibia will tighten up the medial ligament because it slants forward. The tightened medial ligament will then prevent the forward glide of the tibia. Normal and abnormal anterior drawer excursion should thus be eliminated by turning the foot outwards (13.38).

Method

After doing a 90° anterior drawer, the foot is turned out, stabilised, and the anterior drawer repeated. See the sketch (13.39).

Results

A failure to eliminate a positive anterior drawer by external tibial rotation indicates laxity of the medial ligament and medial capsule as well as of the anterior cruciate ligament.

Further evidence of anterior cruciate damage with medial ligament damage would be the demonstration of hyperextension (p. 170), though this also occurs with posterior cruciate ligament injuries.

13.38

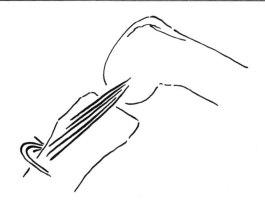

13.39

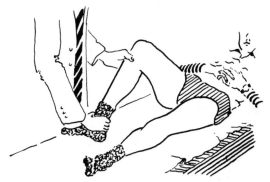

The anterior drawer with internal tibial rotation

Principles

See the principles of the anterior drawer tests, page 148, but briefly: Internal rotation of the tibia tightens up both cruciate ligaments (13.40), so a normal anterior drawer will be eliminated by internal tibial rotation. With a ruptured anterior cruciate, the resulting positive anterior drawer will be eliminated (or at least strongly altered) by internal tibial rotation if the posterior cruciate is intact. This is not because of the direction of the posterior cruciate, which is inappropriate, but because the joint is tightened up, inhibiting the gliding motion. See Slocum & Larson (1968), pp. 217, 219.

Method

Similar to Slocum's test above, but with the foot turned in (13.41).

Results

Failure to eliminate a positive anterior drawer by internal tibial rotation indicates laxity of the posterior cruciate and posterior capsule as well as of the anterior cruciate ligament.

13.40

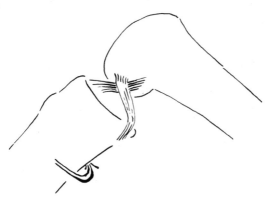

13.41

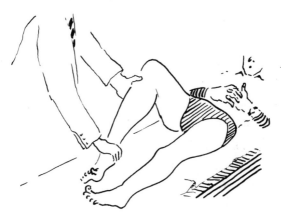

The posterior drawer test

Principles

The posterior cruciate limits posterior glide of the tibial condyle. Its loss should: (i) allow the tibia to drop back; (ii) give an excess of A–P glide. For the former, the appearance of the contour of the knee from the side is crucial. For the latter, it is not easy to distinguish the excessive glide of posterior cruciate deficiency from that of anterior cruciate deficiency.

Method

The knee is first inspected from the lateral side to compare its contour with the other knee. If the tibia appears to be 'dropped back' (see (13.42) and (13.43)), then a positive posterior drawer test is very likely.

A posterior drawer test looks very like an anterior drawer test, the knee being placed at about 80°; see (13.37). The tibia is first gently drawn forwards and the lateral contour checked. It is then firmly pushed back, and the contour inspected critically. Then from the neutral position the tibia is jerked posteriorly, in a to-and-fro manner, looking for excessive 'play'. But as it is difficult to be sure of the neutral starting position, a refinement may be used; see the diagrams.

From a resting position where both knees are at 80°, the suspect leg is lifted (13.44). The patient is asked to lower it slowly (13.45) until it rests in the same position as the other one. At the moment that the muscles relax at the end of the movement, the tibia is seen to drop back (13.46). That confirms a positive posterior drawer test.

Results

Excessive play and knee contour are judged by comparison with the other side, and by experience. A positive posterior drawer test indicates damage to the posterior cruciate ligament and often other posterior capsular structures as well. To confirm damage of this sort one would look also for excessive extension. Theoretically too, any drawer movement should not be controlled by internal rotation, see page 150.

13.42   **13.43**

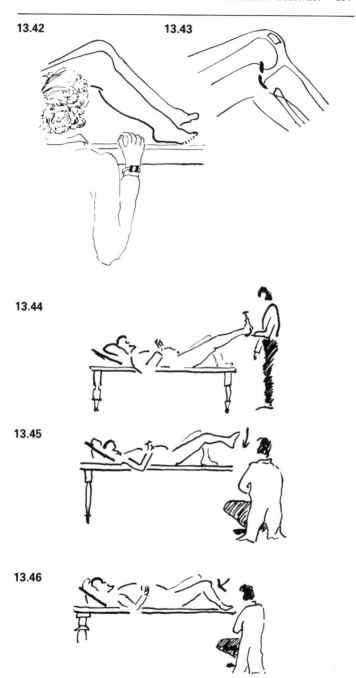

13.44

13.45

13.46

The pivot shift test

Introduction

The pivot shift phenomenon is an alteration in the way the knee moves, caused by lax or torn ligaments. The patient will complain of an unstable knee, and the examiner has to produce that instability clinically, by demonstrating a momentary alteration in the smooth tracking of the joint (13.47). There are many sorts of instability; this test searches for deficiences in one part of the ligamentous support of the knee.

A pivot shift test would never be performed on an acute knee, but in a follow-up clinic. It is not done to see if the knee is stable, but to see what sort of instability there is. A positive result points to laxity of the anterior cruciate and lateral capsule—antero-lateral instability.

The patient will have had a knee injury some time earlier, but will be feeling very unsure of the joint. Painful giving-way, repeated instability when turning while weight-bearing, and instability when decelerating if running are all disabling symptoms to a sportsman. Those symptoms are the indications for this test, and the test should reveal what structures are lax, and therefore whether a certain sort of reconstruction might be successful.

There is a bewildering variety of these tests, not all called a pivot-shift test. There is the MacIntosh test, Slocum's antero-lateral rotary instability test, the jerk test of Hughston et al, and Losee et al's test for anterior subluxation of the lateral tibial plateau. See Losee et al (1978) which gives descriptions and references. All the tests are somewhat alike, but there are good reasons for their differences.

13.47

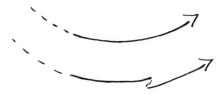

13.48

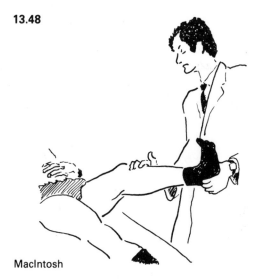

MacIntosh

Principles

Normally as flexion decreases towards extension, the lateral femoral condyle moves smoothly forwards over the lateral tibial plateau, rolling and sliding on its mobile lateral meniscus (13.49). This normal movement is controlled and stabilised by the anterior cruciate and the postero-lateral capsule. The medial femoral condyle is less mobile, sliding rather than rolling as it is stabilised by the powerful deltoid medial ligament upon the more stable medial meniscus (13.50). With the lateral femoral condyle moving back in flexion and forwards in extension there is an element of spin (13.51), a rotary pivot movement that is called conjunct rotation (p. 8).

13.49

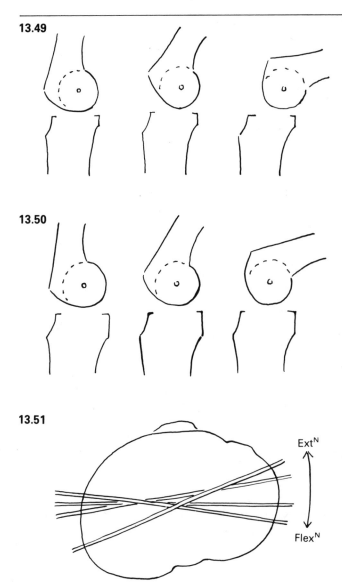

13.50

13.51

Ext^N

Flex^N

In the last part of the movement towards extension, i.e. between 35° flexion and 0°, both cruciates are becoming tensed, the anterior cruciate pulling the lateral femoral condyle forwards, and the posterior cruciate pulling the medial femoral condyle backwards. The result is a rapid increase in conjunct rotation (13.52) as the terminal screw home into close-pack develops. So the femur medially rotates on the tibia if fixed, or the tibia laterally rotates under the femur if fixed. That is what happens normally.

If the anterior cruciate is torn, and there is also damage to the lateral capsule, the unbalanced action of the posterior cruciate may pull both femoral condyles back, or the lateral tibial plateau will sublux anteriorly, as extension is approached (13.53). This abnormal movement may occur with a jerk, and is the basis of the test of Losee (see Losee et al, 1978).

The MacIntosh test has a similar basis, but starts in extension and is produced in the early stages of flexion. Here the lateral tibial plateau starts and remains subluxed anteriorly as flexion begins, but then suddenly reduces backwards at between 20° and 40° of flexion. An exact explanation of this test is more complex (Losee et al, 1978, p. 1028).

The principle of all the tests is that the centre of conjunct rotation (the rotation in the axis of the straight limb) is normally near the middle of the tibial plateau, being around the medial tibial spine (p. 120). With loss or laxity of the anterior cruciate and lateral capsular ligaments, the lateral femoral condyle is 'just waving about in the breeze', free to slip forwards or backwards, uncontrolled by ligaments. The axis of conjunct rotation (pivot) moves suddenly to the medial side (shift), see (13.54).

Slocum's rotary instability test is another pivot shift test based on similar mechanical principles.

13.52

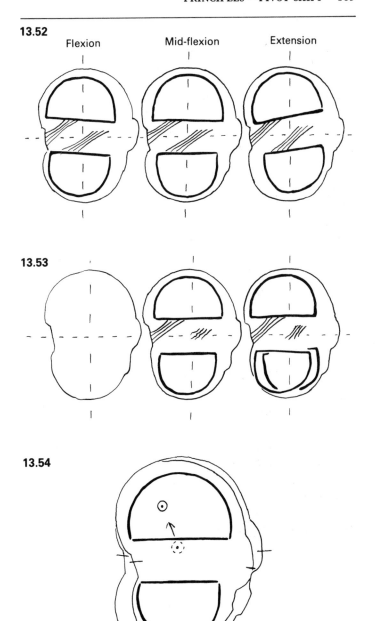

Flexion   Mid-flexion   Extension

13.53

13.54

Method—Losee's test

The patient lies back on a couch. The examiner lifts the limb to be tested, from the same side. For the right leg, he cradles the right ankle against his waist with the leg externally rotated gently. The knee is now lifted, and the whole lower leg is moved proximally, thus relaxing the hamstrings and producing flexion of the knee to about 30°.

Now the left hand is laid on the knee; the thumb pushes the fibular head forwards whilst the fingers pull the patella backwards. Still keeping external rotation with the right hand, a valgus strain is applied by the examiner gently turning to the right whilst holding the lower leg against his abdomen. As the examiner turns, he slowly extends the knee with his left hand, maintaining the thrusts with both hands (13.55). A momentary forward subluxation of the tibial plateau just before extension is reached is a positive result; it should be recognised by the patient as his instability, and felt by the examiner with his left thumb.

Results—Losee's test

A positive test indicates anterior cruciate rupture with postero-lateral capsular damage. The Lachmann's and anterior drawer tests will be found to be positive also; and the varus stress test. Some say this test is a little too sensitive. There are some caveats (see Losee, 1978).

Method—MacIntosh's lateral pivot shift test (MacIntosh, 1972)

The patient lies back on a couch. The examiner lifts the limb to be tested from the same side. For the right leg, he holds it at the heel with an internal rotation stress, and the knee in extension. Now the knee is gently flexed by the left hand (13.56 and 13.57). A sudden anterior shift of the lateral tibial plateau (caused by the internal rotation pressure of the right hand) is a positive result.

13.55

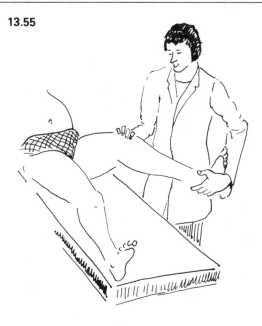

13.56

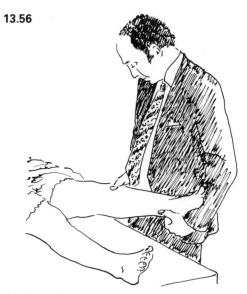

MacIntosh's

Results—MacIntosh's test

As with Losee's test, a positive result indicates anterior cruciate rupture with postero-lateral damage. There should also be a positive Lachmann's and anterior drawer test, and a positive varus stress test, even in extension.

Method—Slocum's antero-lateral rotary instability test (Slocum et al, 1976)

For the right knee, the patient lies on his left side with hips and knees slightly flexed, say 30°. The examiner stands behind the patient. The patient tilts the pelvis towards the examiner some 30° or more, and places his right foot on the couch just behind the left foot. See (13.58)

Now the examiner lays his hands on the right knee. Pressing down very slightly to exert a varus force, he rocks the knee backwards into extension and then forwards again into flexion. A positive test may be seen and felt—a sudden movement of the lateral tibial condyle occurring typically as the knee first flexes from the extended position.

This test exerts the same stresses as the MacIntosh test. The instep of the foot, resting on the couch, is internally rotated with respect to the backward tilted pelvis; the knee hangs between hip and foot and so has a valgus strain on it. This is the preferred test if the patient cannot relax easily or if the limb is large and difficult to grasp.

Results—Slocum's test

If positive, Slocum's antero-lateral test indicates the same as MacIntosh's and Losee's test—anterior cruciate rupture plus postero-lateral laxity. The anterior drawer tests should also be positive, and the varus stress test too, even in extension (see recurvatum test, below).

Method—the 'jerk' test of Hughston et al

This is written up in Hughston et al (1976), pp. 164–165. It may be less reliable than the others.

13.57

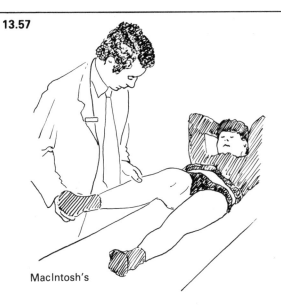

MacIntosh's

13.58

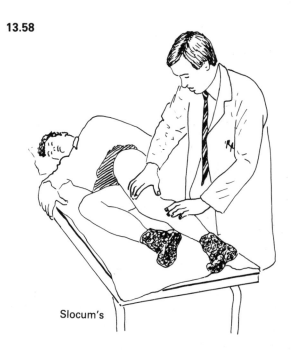

Slocum's

The check for excessive extension, or the recurvatum test

Principles

When the knee is straight, further extension is prevented by the rising tension in the ligaments, caused by the separation of their bony attachments, in turn caused by the mechanics of the joint—the cam effect of the femoral condyle, and axial rotation etc. The joint surfaces are thrust together as the ligaments are tensed, till extensor movement is stopped. If ligaments become torn or lax, or if loss of articular surface decreases the distance between their bony attachments, the extensor motion will be stopped later, i.e. there will be excessive extension.

Method

Light palmar pressure holds the knee joint to the couch, while the other hand lifts the foot by the big toe. This method allows rapid comparison between left and right. There are other methods, see opposite.

Results

It is unusual for normal extension to be more than 5°. Excluding adults with generalised joint laxity and girls with growth problems, extension may be excessive in a joint with serious multiple ligament laxity, often of anterior cruciate and medial ligament.

But this test is not at all specific. It only says 'this joint is pathologically lax'. Ballet dancers may develop genu recurvatum from forcing the knee back when 'up on points', and patients with severe quadriceps weakness similarly from locking the knee into extension in stance phase to prevent the joint from giving way under the body weight.

A recurvatum test in external rotation is described in Hughston et al (1976) on page 165. The external rotation should prevent any recurvatum if the medial complex is intact.

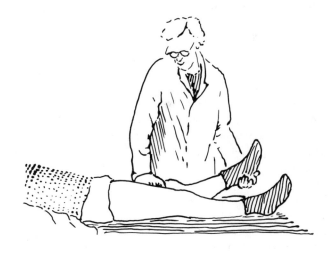

Tests for cartilage damage

Principles

If the femoral condyles are moved across a raised meniscal fragment, they produce a 'click'. See (13.59) and (13.60). This or other meniscal damage such as a circumferential tear (13.61) may also produce pain. This painful click can be accentuated if the femoral and tibial condyles are forced together, thus putting a squeeze on the menisci.

The production of a painful click, or even just pain, under such conditions points towards meniscus injury, though the test is not entirely reliable. The click might for instance come from a normal meniscus moving over degenerated articular cartilage. Also the click must come *from the joint line*, and not, for example, from tendons around the joint.

A simple manoeuvre, based on the anatomy of the joint, can put a squeeze on the meniscus. Thus external rotation of the tibia, acting through the forward angulation of the medial ligament, will draw the medial tibial condyle up against the femur and so cause compression of the medial meniscus (13.62, 13.65). Similarily, because the lateral ligament angles forward in flexion, internal tibial rotation in flexion will tighten the lateral compartment, and compress the lateral meniscus (13.63, 13.65).

In a McMurray's test, from the fully flexed position and with one or the other forced rotation, the joint is slowly extended while the tips of the fingers press in on the relevant side of the joint line. This fingerwork ensures greater pressure on the meniscus and accurate localisation of any click. The examiner's eyes watch the patient's face for pain signals.

Here is a quotation from *A Practice of Orthopoedic Surgery* by McMurray (1946).

> With the alteration of the angle of the joint [towards extension from full flexion] any loose portion of the internal cartilage is caught between the articular surfaces of the femur and the tibia, and the sliding of the femur over the the abnormal portion of the cartilage is accompanied by an appreciable click and pain, which the patient states is the same as he already experiences when the knee gives way.

These are the general principles for posterior lesions of the menisci, applying to McMurray's manoeuvre and Apley's grinding test (Apley, 1947).

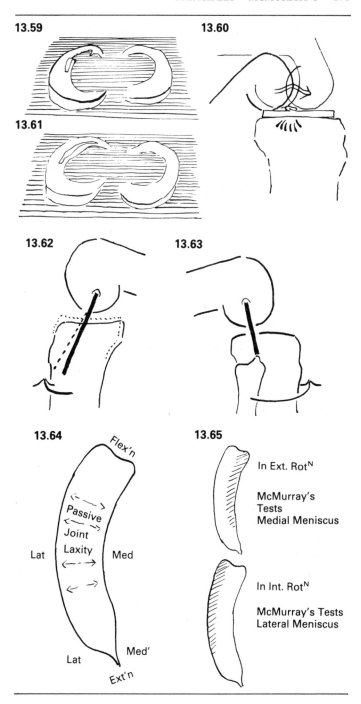

13.59

13.60

13.61

13.62

13.63

13.64

Flex'n

Passive

Joint

Laxity

Lat   Med

Lat

Med'

Ext'n

13.65

In Ext. Rot^N

McMurray's
Tests
Medial Meniscus

In Int. Rot^N

McMurray's Tests
Lateral Meniscus

When the lesion is anterior the joint line is more accessible: direct pressure on either the antero-medial or the antero-lateral aspect of the joint, while slowly extending from about 90°, may elicit the pain or a click.

Method

The foot is grasped either anteriorly on the tarsus or underneath by the heel. The knee is put into full flexion by approaching the foot to the buttock. For the medial meniscus the foot is turned outwards while the fingers compress the postero-medial joint line; see (13.66). Using the leg as a lever arm and holding the foot turned out, the knee is gently extended. The fingers on the knee feel for the joint line clicks and the eyes watch the patient's face. This is the usual form of McMurray's test.

Modifications of McMurray's test are usually in the form of repeated scooping movements instead of a smooth continuous movement. For the posterior horn of the medial meniscus the knee is in full flexion, the leg is turned into external rotation, and the heel is scooped around the medial and lateral quadrants of full flexion. See (13.67). The same is done with the leg in internal rotation for a posterior horn of the lateral meniscus. The knee hand should palpate deeply the appropriate side of the posterior joint line. This scooping motion can be repeated in different degrees of extension, as progressively more anterior parts of the meniscus are searched for injury. See (13.68).

Results

The results of the examination must be taken together with an appropriate history—of giving way, locking, or of recurrent effusions. The presence of a click or clunk in the joint line, especially if painful, suggests meniscal damage. But painful clicks can occur all round the knee, from tendons flicking over protuberances or from uneven rubbing between fascial planes. These should be distinguished by locating the fingers accurately on the joint line, but it is not always easy to be sure. The diagnosis of meniscus injury is never certain clinically, not the location, nor even which side is involved. With the advent of endoscopy, the summary after a positive result tends to be: 'This may well be a meniscus injury, but requires arthroscopy, and maybe arthroscopic surgery'.

13.66

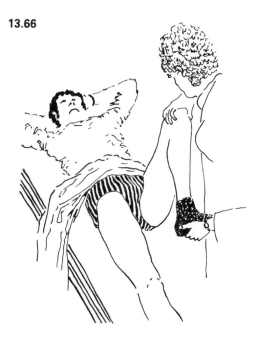

13.67 Flexion

13.68

Extension

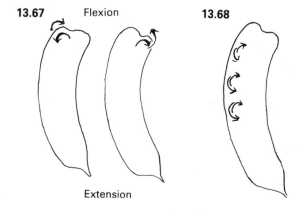

Bibliography

Akerblom B 1948 Standing and sitting posture. Nordiska Bokhandeln, Stockholm

Apley A G 1947 The diagnosis of meniscus injuries—some new clinical methods. Journal of Bone and Joint Surgery 29: 78–84

Austin R T 1981 Photostreptograph of patellar tracking. Injury 13: 260–261

Barnett C H 1953 Locking at the knee joint. Journal of Anatomy 87: 91–95

Barnett C H, Richardson A T 1953 The postural function of the popliteus muscle. Annals of Physical Medicine 1: 177–179

Brantigan O C, Voshell A F 1941 The mechanics of the ligaments and menisci of the knee joint. Journal of Bone and Joint Surgery 23 (1): 44–66

Brantigan O C, Voshell A F 1943 The tibial collateral ligament: Its function, its bursae, and its relationship to the medial meniscus. Journal of Bone and Joint Surgery 25 (1): 121–131

Bullough P G, Goodfellow J, O'Connor J 1973 The relationship between degenerative changes and loadbearing in the human hip. Journal of Bone and Joint Surgery 55-B:746

Danzig L A, Newell J D, Guerra J, Resnick D 1981 Osseous landmarks of the normal knee. Clinical Orthopaedics 156: 201–206

De peretti F, Lacroix R, Bourgeon A, Argenson C, Richelme H 1983 Geometry of the facies articularis superior tibiae and rotation of the knee. Anatomica Clinica 5: 3–7

Evans P J 1979 The postural function of the iliotibial tract. Annals of the Royal College of Surgeons (England) 61: 271–280

Evans P J 1985 Postural uses of the close-packed condition of joints. Annals of the Royal College of Surgeons (England) 67(1): 53

Fairbank T J 1948 knee joint changes after menisectomy. Journal of Bone and Joint Surgery 30-B (4): 664–670

Ficat R P, Hungerford D S 1977 Disorders of the patello-femoral joint. Masson, Paris; Williams Wilkins, Baltimore

Furman W, Marshall J L, Girgis F G 1976 The anterior cruciate ligament. Journal of Bone and Joint Surgery 58-A: 179–185

Girgis F G, Marshall J L, Monajem A R S 1975 The cruciate ligaments of the knee joint. Clinical Orthopaedics 106: 216–231

Glasgow M, McClelland C J, Campbell J, Jackson R W 1981 The Synovial plica and its significance in the knee. Journal of Bone and Joint Surgery 63-B: 630

Goodfellow J, Hungerford D S, Zindel M 1976a Patello-femoral joint mechanics and pathology 1. Functional anatomy of the patello-femoral joint. Journal of Bone and Joint Surgery 58-B (3): 287–290

Goodfellow J, Hungerford D S, Woods C 1976b Patello-femoral joint mechanics and pathology 2. Chondromalacia patellae. Journal of Bone and Joint Surgery 58-B (3): 291–299

Guymer J 1984 Clinical Tutor in Physiotherapy, Westminster Hospital, London. Personal communication.

Hoffa A 1904 The influence of the adipose tissue with regard to the pathology of the knee joint. Journal of the American Medical Association 43: 795–796

Hseih H, Walker P S 1976 Stabilising mechanisms of the loaded and unloaded knee Joint. Journal of Bone and Joint Surgery 58-A (1): 87–93

Hughston J C, Andrews J R, Cross M J, Moschi A 1976 Classification of knee ligament instabilities Part 1. The medial compartment and cruciate ligaments. Journal of Bone and Joint Surgery 58-A: 159–172

Hughston J C, Andrews J R, Cross M J, Moschi A 1976 Classification of knee ligament instabilities Part 2. The lateral compartment. Journal of Bone and Joint Surgery 58-A: 173–179.

Hungerford D S, Barry M 1979 Biomechanics of the patello-femoral joint. Clin Orthopoedics 144: 9–15

Insall J 1982 Patellar pain. Journal of Bone and Joint Surgery 64-A (1): 147–152

Jeffreys T E 1963 Recurrent dislocation of the patella due to abnormal attachment of the iliotibial tract. Journal of Bone and Joint Surgery 45-B: 740–743.

Kaplan E B 1956 The lateral menisco-femoral ligament of the knee joint. Bulletin of the Hospital for Joint Diseases 17: 176–181

Kettlecamp D B 1981 Management of patellar malalignment. Journal of Bone and Joint Surgery 63-A (8): 1344–1347

Last R J 1948 Some anatomical details of the knee joint. Journal of Bone and Joint Surgery 30-B (4): 683–688

Last R J 1950 The popliteus muscle and the lateral meniscus. Journal of Bone and Joint Surgery 32-B (1): 93–99

Levens A S, Inman V T 1948 Transverse rotation of the segments of the lower extremity in locomotion. Journal of Bone and Joint Surgery 30-A (4) 859–872

Losee R E, Johnson T R, Southwick W O 1978 Anterior subluxation of the lateral tibial plateau. Journal of Bone and Joint Surgery 60-A (8): 1015–1030

MacConaill M A 1932 The function of intra-articular fibrocartilages, with special reference to the knee and inferior radio-ulnar joints. Journal of Anatomy 66: 210–227

MacConaill M A 1953 The movement of bones and joints and the significance of shape. Journal of Bone and Joint Surgery 35-B (2): 290–297

MacConaill M A 1964 Joint movement. Physiotherapy Nov 1964: 359–367

MacConaill M A, Basmajian J V 1977 Muscles and movements. Robert E Kreiger Publishing Company, Huntingdon, New York

MacIntosh D L 1972 Pivot shift—a clinical sign of symptomatic anterior cruciate insufficiency. Journal of Bone and Joint Surgery 54-B: 743

McMurray T P 1946 A practice of orthopaedic surgery. Edward Arnold and Co, London

McRae R 1983 Clinical orthopaedic examination, 2nd edn. Churchill Livingstone, Edinburgh

Markolf K L, Mensch J S, Amstutz H C 1976 Stiffness and laxity of the knee—the contribution of the supporting structures. Journal of Bone and Joint Surgery 58-A (5): 583–593

Noyes F R, Grood E S 1976 The strength of the anterior cruciate ligament in humans and rhesus monkeys. Journal of Bone and joint Surgery 58-A (8): 1074–1082

Ober F R 1935 slipping patella or recurrent dislocation of the patella. Journal of Bone and Joint Surgery 17(3): 774–779

Ober F R 1936 Role of the iliotibial band and fascia lata as a factor in the causation of low back disabilities and sciatica. Journal of Bone and Joint Surgery 18: 105–110

O'Donoghue D H 1950 Surgical treatment of fresh injuries to the major ligaments of the knee. Journal of Bone and Joint Surgery 32-A (4): 721–731

Phillips H 1984 Orthopoedic Surgeon, Norfolk and Norwich Hospital, England. Personal communication.

Pipkin G 1971 Knee injuries: The role of the suprapatellar plica and suprapatellar bursa in simulating internal derangements. Clinical Orthopaedics 74: 161–174

Radin E L, Paul I L 1972 A consolidated concept of joint lubrication. Journal of Bone and Joint Surgery 54-A (3): 607–616

Saunders J B deC M, Inman V T, Eberhart H D 1953 The major determinants in normal and pathological gait. Journal of Bone and Joint Surgery 35-A (3): 543–558

Seebacher J R, Inglis A E, Marshall J L, Warren R F 1982 The structure of the postero-lateral aspect of the knee. Journal of Bone and Joint Surgery 64-A (4): 536–541

Seedhom B 1976 The loadbearing function of the menisci. Physiotherapy 62 (7): 223–226.

Slocum D B, Larson R L 1968 Rotatory instability of the knee. Journal of Bone and Joint Surgery 50-A (2): 211–225

Slocum D B, James S L, Larson R L, Singer K M 1976 Clinical test for anterolateral rotary instability of the knee. Clinical Orthopaedics 118: 63–69

Smillie I S 1948 The congenital discoid meniscus. Journal of Bone and Joint Surgery 30-B (4): 671–682

Smith J W 1953 The act of standing. Acta Orthopaedica Scandinavica 23: 159–168

Smith J W 1956 Observations on the postural mechanisms of the human knee joint. Journal of Anatomy 90: 236–290

Stickland A 1984 Examination of the knee Joint. Physiotherapy 70 (4): 144–150

Stoker D J 1980 Knee arthrography. Chapman and Hall, London

Struben P J 1982 The tibial plateau. Journal of Bone and Joint Surgery 64-B (3): 336–339

Trent P S, Walker P S, Wolf B 1976 Ligament length patterns, strength, and rotational axes of the knee joint. Clinical Orthopaedics 117: 263–270

Trickey E L 1982 Pathological anatomy of knee joint injuries. In: Helfet A J (ed) Disorders of the knee. Lippincott, Philiadelphia

Walker P S, Hajek J V 1972 The loadbearing area in the knee joint. Journal of Biomechanics 5: 581–589.

Warren L F, Girgis F G 1974 The prime static stabiliser of the medial side of the knee. Journal of Bone and Joint Surgery 56-A (4): 665–674

Wyke B D 1967 The neurology of joints. Annals of the Royal College of Surgeons (England) 41: 25–50.

Wyke B D 1972 Articular neurology—a review. Physiotherapy 58 (3): 94

Wynne-Davies R 1970 Acetabular dysplasia and familial joint laxity: Two etiological factors in congenital dislocation of the hip. A review of 589 patients and their families. Journal of Bone and Joint Surgery 52-B: 704–716

Glossary

Apophysis. Clinical term for a centre of ossification (epiphysis) at the site of insertion of a large muscle; examples are the tibial tuberosity and the heel. A traction epiphysis.

Apophysitis. Inflammation of a traction epiphysis, probably stress-related.

Arthritis. Affliction of a joint; properly, inflammation in a joint. Many sorts, e.g. rheumatoid, osteo., septic, sterile, gouty, haemophilic.

Arthrography. Double-contrast (air + medium) X-ray of a joint. Reveals the surfaces of internal structures such as menisci, and capsular defects.

Arthrodesis. Elimination of a joint, with bony union between the two bones. (Latin desistere = to end, desist, discontinue.)

Arthroplasty. Literally, the fashioning of a joint. Joint replacement, with the removal of the whole joint, as in the hip (total hip), or by surface replacement as in the knee.

Arthroscopy. Looking inside a joint through a joint endoscope.

Arthrotomy. Cutting open a joint (surgically).

Aspiration. Withdrawing fluid (either effusion or haemarthrosis) from a joint cavity through a needle. Paracentesis.

Baker's cyst. A popliteal cyst caused by rupture of the posterior capsule of the knee joint, with herniation of synovium.

Bone, accessory. Small, occasional bone. There are a number of these ossicles in the foot, usually representing bones that were present in earlier evolutionary forms, e.g. the os trigonum.

Bone, sesamoid. Bone like a sesame seed. Found in tendons near joints, often inconstantly. The fabella may be palpable and visible on X-ray, or absent. The patella is a large sesamoid bone.

Bucket handle tear, of meniscus. A tear parallel to the outer meniscal margin. The inner free edge splits off, becomes pushed centrally by the articulating femoral condyle, but still remains attached front and back like a bucket handle.

Bursitis. Inflammation of a bursa, often from trauma or over-use. Often occupational, such as house-maid's knee, now more often seen in carpet-layers. Occasionally infective.

Calcification. In medial ligament, see Pellegrini-Steida disease. In menisci, called chondrocalcinosis (not covered here).

Chondromalacia. A degradation of articular cartilage, with many theories to account for it, see Goodfellow (1976). Sometimes used as a diagnostic label for patello-femoral pain of unknown cause.

Close-pack. State found at one end of joint range, when the articular surfaces are most congruent, most ligaments are taut, and the intra-synovial volume is least.

Condyle. Enlarged, rounded end of a long bone which articulates with another bone. From the Greek word meaning knuckle.

Cyst, Baker's. See Baker's cyst.

Cyst, popliteal. A herniation of synovium through the posterior capsule of the knee joint, causing a swelling in the popliteal fossa. Frequently secondary to a persistent joint effusion.

Diaphysis. That part of a growing long bone derived from the primary ossification centre. Shaft of growing bone.

Dislocation. Total separation of joint surfaces. Recurrent dislocation happens often; habitual dislocation happens always. Compare subluxation, q.v.

Effusion, joint. Exudate in a joint, either traumatic or inflammatory.

Epicondyle. Pit or knob on the side of a condyle. Usually sited on the axis of hinge movement in flexion.

Epiphysiolysis. Ablation (lysis) of a cartilaginous growth plate (epiphyseal plate), e.g. by staples that span across it.

Epiphysis. Extremity of a growing long bone, developed from a secondary ossification centre, and separated from the shaft by an epiphyseal plate—the cartilage growth plate. Also used loosely to describe the growth plate itself. A *pressure* epiphysis forms part of a joint; a *traction* epiphysis develops at the attachment of a powerful muscle; *atavistic* epiphyses occur at sites where in earlier evolution separate skeletal elements were present.

Excision arthroplasty. Cutting out a joint and replacing it with an artificial joint.

Fabella. Small sesamoid bone found where the lateral head of gastrocnemius rubs on the lateral femoral condyle in extension. Inconstant. Size is 2–4 mm on X-ray.

Facet. Mark on bone, depressed or raised, where collagen of ligament or tendon attaches, for example, posterior cruciate. Occasionally for articulation.

Fibrillation. Fine cracking of the surface of articular cartilage.

Fixed length. Term used for structures made of collagen or scar tissue (length does not change) rather than muscle (contractile), especially where they cross two joints, so that a change in the position of the proximal joint will cause an effect at the attachment beyond the distal joint. The iliotibial tract and the plantar fascia produce *physiological* fixed length phenomena; Volkmann's ischaemic contracture produces *pathological* ditto in the forearm.

Friction syndrome. A painful rubbing between tissue planes or over bony prominences, usually experienced by athletes who are over-keen or undertrained, as in charity marathons. Can also occur in industry with job changes, e.g. tenosynovitis at the wrist. See also over-use syndrome.

Genu valgum. Knock knee.

Genu varum. Bow leg.

Haemarthrosis. Blood in a joint. A joint swelling immediately after an injury (say within two hours) is usually blood; especially if very tense and very painful, with much muscle spasm.

Horizontal tear of meniscus. A split parallel to the tibial plateau.

I.D.K. Internal derangement of the knee. Used of an acute knee that is too swollen and too painful to examine properly, when the history and the examination point to a substantial injury.

Joint space. The space between the bones of a joint on an X-ray. Considered to be a measure of articular cartilage thickness, especially if weight-bearing.

Jumper's knee. Pain at the inferior pole of the patella, an over-use syndrome (q.v.). Repeated small avulsions, with repeated attempts at healing.

Laxity. Looseness, mechanical play in a joint, usually in accessory movements such as passive glides or rotations, or varus/valgus movements. Some laxity is normal in loose-pack. Excessive laxity is judged by experience and by comparison with the other side.

Lipping. Bony build-up, producing a spike or lip of bone. Found at the margins of the joint surfaces in osteo-arthritis; also from calcification of repeatedly strained ligament or capsule in sport. See also osteophyte.

Loose body. Freely movable fragment inside joint, usually visible on X-ray. May be from osteochondritis dissecans (q.v), or from a detached osteophyte in osteo-arthritis.

Loose-pack. Majority of range of joint movement, where there is normally some laxity of accessory movements. Opposite of close-pack (q.v).

Manipulation. In physiotherapy: highly specific gentle graded movements (mobilisations) of one bone; may reduce pain by their effect on contracted collagen or by influencing neurological afferent impulses. In osteoopathy: rapid, short-range movement, to 'put the joint back'. In surgery: movement of grossly stiffened joint designed to break down adhesion; usually under general anaesthesia.

Metaphysis. That part of the diapysis (shaft) of a growing long bone that is adjacent to the epiphyseal cartilage. The place where a diaphysis is actively growing.

Osgood-Schlatter's disease. An apophysitis, with pain and swelling at the tibial tubercle. Chronic strain or over-use at the site of pull of the patellar tendon causes the epiphysis (apophysis) to separate slightly at the cartilage plate.

Osteo-arthritis. Degenerative disease of joints, with loss of articular cartilage and lipping. Often follows trauma or other disease. May be painful.

Osteo-arthropathy. Bony pathology in a joint. Charcot's osteo-arthropathy is a gross destruction of the joint that follows loss of proprioceptive sensation in that joint, sometimes from siphylis affecting the posterior columns of the spinal cord.

Osteochondral fracture. Fracture of bone and cartilate, i.e. involving the joint surface. Must produce haemarthrosis, probably with fat globules in it.

Osteochondritis. Literally, inflammation at junction of cartilage and bone, but not always so. In osteochondritis juvenalis, there is necrosis and softening of a bony epiphysis. Examples are in the head of the femur (Perthes' disease), and the navicular bone (Kohler's disease). In osteochondritis dissecans (literally the cutting apart of bone and cartilage), a piece of cartilage with underlying bone loosens from a joint surface, and may become detached and form a loose body in the knee. Osgood-Schlatter's disease may be called an osteochondritis, but is a traumatic apophysitis.

Osteophyte. Literally 'bony plant (growth)'. Spur or beak of bone appearing to have grown, often from a joint margin or at the attachment of a ligament.

Osteotomy. Cutting a bone, then allowing it to heal in a different orientation, thus altering the force transmission through a painful joint. Also for malalignment or leg length discrepancy.

Over-use syndromes. From sports medicine or industry. Pain where fascial planes rub across each other, or at the sites of bursae, where lubrication has been inadequate; or pain at the site of repeated avulsions where collagen is attached to bone. Example of the former, iliotibial tract friction syndrome; of the latter, jumper's knee, tennis elbow.

Paracentesis. See aspiration.

Parrot-beak tear of meniscus. Folded-over tag caused by split in meniscal cartilage.

Pedunculated tear of meniscus. Tear from the (inner) free edge into a meniscus, and then (for example) backwards circumferentially towards the posterior horn, leaving a free pedunculated tag.

Pellegrini-Steida disease. Development of ossification at site of upper attachment of medial complex of knee. Pain after injury, with subsequent formation of an osteophyte in the resulting haematoma.

Recurvatum, (genu) recurvatum. (Knee) bent backwards, hyper-extended.

Rheumatoid arthritis. Pain, stiffness and swelling of synovial joints, often with over-growth of synovium and erosion and loss of articular cartilage. May cause marked deformity in hands and knees.

Snapping knee. Affliction with many causes, either inside the joint (e.g. meniscus), or outside the joint (fibrous thickenings flicking across protuberances).

Soft tissue injury. Injury of joint that does not shown up on an X-ray, i.e. damage to muscle, tendon, ligament, capsule, &c.

Stance phase. Applying to one leg in walking, period when that leg is weight-bearing. Extends from heel-strike to toe-off.

Strain. Partial tear of a ligament or muscle, usually not impairing power or stability when healed.

Stress disorder. See over-use syndrome.

Sub-chondral. (Directly) beneath articular cartilage.

Sublux, Subluxation. Displacement of articular surfaces so that they are still in partial contact. Compare dislocation, q.v.

Surface replacement. In joint replacement, replacing the articular surface of a joint (e.g. tibial component of knee), rather than the whole joint (e.g. hip).

Swing phase. The period in walking when the leg is off the ground, non-weightbearing, swinging forwards.

Trochlea. Greek, meaning 'pulley'. Saddle-shaped part of bone, like a section of a pulley. Of femur, of talus, and of humerus.

Tubercle. Literally, a little lump, usually on a bone.

Valgus. With distal portion deviating outwards.

Varus. With distal portion deviating inwards.

Windswept deformity. With one knee varus and one knee valgus, as if blown thus by a wind from one side.

Index